Heartburn & Reflux

FOR

DUMMIES®

by Carol Ann Rinzler
with Ken DeVault, MD

WILEY
Wiley Publishing, Inc.

Heartburn & Reflux For Dummies®

Published by
Wiley Publishing, Inc.
111 River St.
Hoboken, NJ 07030-5774
www.wiley.com

For general information on our other products and services or to obtain technical support, please contact our Customer Care Department within the U.S. at 800-762-2974, outside the U.S. at 317-572-3993, or fax 317-572-4002.

Wiley also publishes its books in a variety of electronic formats. Some content that appears in print may not be available in electronic books.

Library of Congress Control Number: 2004103167

ISBN: 978-0-7645-5688-3

Manufactured in the United States of America

20 19 18 17 16 15 14 13 12 11 10 9 8 7 6 5

1O/RW/QW/QU/IN

About the Author

Carol Ann Rinzler is a noted authority on health and nutrition and holds an MA from Columbia University. She writes a weekly nutrition column for the *New York Daily News* and is the author of more than 20 health-related books including *Nutrition For Dummies, Controlling Cholesterol For Dummies, Weight Loss Kit For Dummies,* and the highly acclaimed *Estrogen and Breast Cancer: A Warning to Women.* Rinzler lives in New York with her husband, wine writer Perry Luntz, and their amiable cat, Kat.

About the Contributor and Medical Consultant

Ken DeVault, MD is a Professor of Medicine and has been active in research and education in the area of gastroesophageal reflux disease (GERD) for over 20 years. Dr. DeVault conducts research on topics that include the acute and chronic treatment of gastroesophageal reflux, Barrett's Esophagus, and esophageal motility. He has a particular interest in esophageal diseases in an aging population. Publishing extensively since the late 1980s, Dr. DeVault has written over 150 book chapters, abstracts, editorials, and original articles. He is the co-author of the American College of Gastroenterology's Guideline Statement on GERD, which is now in its third edition.

Dr. DeVault received his undergraduate degree from the University of Tennessee and his medical degree from the Bowman Gray School of Medicine at Wake Forest University. He completed his internship and residency in internal medicine at Vanderbilt University and completed a combined clinical and research fellowship at Jefferson Medical College in Philadelphia, PA. He is a Trustee and Fellow of the American College of Gastroenterology and serves on committees of the American College of Gastroenterology, American Gastroenterological Association, and American Society of Gastrointestinal Endoscopy.

Dedication

For my husband, Perry Luntz.

Author's Acknowledgments

This new project of *Heartburn & Reflux For Dummies* has given me the opportunity to work with yet another group of thoroughly pleasant professionals at the *For Dummies* group at Wiley Publishing, Inc. Acquisitions Editor Natasha Graf was a joy to work with as were Project Editor Mike Baker and Copy Editor Chad Sievers. I'm truly indebted to Ken DeVault for his careful and valuable comments on the medical aspects of this book. One is lucky indeed to find such as skillful contributor. I also thank Robert Rakel for serving as the technical reviewer. I also am grateful to the National Heartburn Alliance for their help during this project.

Publisher's Acknowledgments

We're proud of this book; please send us your comments through our Dummies online registration form located at www.dummies.com/register/.

Some of the people who helped bring this book to market include the following:

Acquisitions, Editorial, and Media Development

Project Editor: Mike Baker

Acquisitions Editor: Natasha Graf

Copy Editor: Chad Sievers

Technical Reviewer: Robert Rakel, MD

Editorial Manager: Jennifer Ehrlich

Editorial Assistants: Courtney Allen, Elizabeth Rea

Cover Photos: © PHOTOTAKE Inc./Alamy

Cartoons: Rich Tennant, www.the5thwave.com

Composition

Project Coordinator: Maridee Ennis

Layout and Graphics: Andrea Dahl, Denny Hager, Stephanie D. Jumper, Brent Savage, Jacque Schneider, Janet Seib, Mary Gillot Virgin

Special Art: Kathryn Born

Proofreaders: Andy Hollandbeck, Carl Pierce, Dwight Ramsey, Brian Walls, TECHBOOKS Production Services

Indexer: TECHBOOKS Production Services

Special Help

Christina Guthrie, Natalie F. Harris, Laura Miller

Publishing and Editorial for Consumer Dummies

Diane Graves Steele, Vice President and Publisher, Consumer Dummies

Joyce Pepple, Acquisitions Director, Consumer Dummies

Kristin A. Cocks, Product Development Director, Consumer Dummies

Michael Spring, Vice President and Publisher, Travel

Brice Gosnell, Associate Publisher, Travel

Kelly Regan, Editorial Director, Travel

Publishing for Technology Dummies

Andy Cummings, Vice President and Publisher, Dummies Technology/General User

Composition Services

Gerry Fahey, Vice President of Production Services

Debbie Stailey, Director of Composition Services

Contents at a Glance

Table of Contents

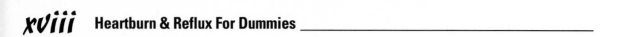

Introduction

· ·

*H*eartburn is a pain. When you have heartburn, eating the food you like best, working at top speed, or enjoying activities with your family, friends, and significant others can be difficult. That's the bad news.

But heartburn can be helped. You have all sorts of options: Carefully editing your diet, eating smaller meals, loosening your belt, or working with your doctor to find effective medicine can help you to eat the foods you like, work at top speed, and yes, enjoy extracurricular activities with family, friends, and significant others. That's the good news.

The great news is that *Heartburn & Reflux For Dummies* spells it all out.

About This Book

Heartburn & Reflux For Dummies isn't a medical textbook, so you don't have to go to medical school or be a science wiz in order to get through it. Instead, the book aims to give you — in an easily digestible form — the information that you need to make sensible choices about how to handle that annoying pain in your middle.

More than 60 million Americans experience heartburn every year, but that doesn't mean they're all experts on the subject. For readers who know absolutely nothing about heartburn except that it hurts, I offer basic definitions and explanations in this book. For those of you who know more than a little about heartburn, this book is both a refresher course and a guide to the latest skinny on reflux. For everyone, this book is packed with nuggets of fascinating stuff like the biography of the man who invented heartburn surgery and a quiz on movies about babies. (In the chapter on infants with heartburn, of course.)

My goal is to help you recognize and treat a condition that may range from simply annoying to unpleasantly painful to potentially hazardous to your overall health. Giving you the ammo you need to soothe your aching middle and prevent future complications means laying out the facts and then sticking in a bit of air (like that movie quiz) so you can take a deep breath and move on to even more facts — like how to live a happy, healthy life even if Mother Nature tosses heartburn in your path.

This book is a great guide to understanding and handling heartburn, reflux, and gastroesophageal reflux disease (GERD). But you don't have to stop here. I provide you with all kinds of additional sources for assistance that you can use your phone, modem, and mail carrier to access.

Please note that the material in this book is for your information only. When it comes to medical advice, your most certain guide is your doctor, the person most familiar with your health and your medical needs. In addition, except where specifically noted, the material in this book applies to adults.

Conventions Used in This Book

To help you navigate your way through this book, I use the following conventions:

- ✔ *Italic* is used for emphasis and to highlight new words or terms that are defined.
- ✔ **Boldfaced** text is used to indicate keywords in bulleted lists or the action part of numbered steps.
- ✔ `Monofont` is used for Web addresses.

One more thing: I provide you with tons of Web sites in this book that you can use to get *even more* information on various heartburn-related topics. But, nowadays, Web addresses seem to have the shelf life of freshly baked bread. They can be great one day and stale the next. So, if you happen to find a specific address in this book that they've changed on us, I suggest scaling it back by going to the main site — the part of the address that ends in .com, .org, or .edu — and snooping around a bit.

What You're Not to Read

Yes, you read that right. You don't have to read every single word I've written here. Some small parts of this title are fun and informative but not necessarily vital to your understanding of heartburn.

- ✔ **Text in sidebars:** Sidebars, which look like text enclosed in a shaded gray box, appear here and there throughout the book. I like them, and I think you will too, but your functional knowledge of heartburn won't be adversely affected should you walk on by.
- ✔ **Anything accompanied by a Technical Stuff icon:** This info is good (really good) but not critical to getting a handle on heartburn.

> ✔ **The barcodes on the back of the book:** I'm not sure who put those there, but I know that I didn't. So, you have my permission not to read them.

Foolish Assumptions

Every book is written with a particular reader in mind, and this one is no different. As I wrote it, I made the following basic assumptions about who you are and why you plunked down your hard-earned cash for a 300+ page book about heartburn.

> ✔ You don't have a medical degree, but you've decided it would be smart to know more about why you hurt.
>
> ✔ You've changed your diet and tried all the antiheartburn drugs you can get without a prescription, and now you think it's time to figure out where to go for serious advice.
>
> ✔ You want basic information about heartburn, the people who treat it, and the medicines that relieve it.
>
> ✔ You've been recently diagnosed with heartburn or acid reflux disease or think you may have it.

How This Book Is Organized

The following is a brief summary of each part in *Heartburn & Reflux For Dummies.* You can use this information as a "quick pick" guide to check out what you want to read first.

Part 1: Naming Your Pain

In Chapter 1, I give you an overview of practically everything you need to know about heartburn, including stats on how many of your fellow citizens are in the Heartburn Boat with you. Chapter 2 presents a really clear guide to your digestive organs — including the ones that hurt when heartburn hits. In Chapter 3, I list heartburn's symptoms and (sorry about this) the potential consequences. And I reserve Chapter 4 for naming names — telling you who's at risk, and why.

Part II: Eating Your Way to Relief

I start this part by covering nutrition in Chapter 5, telling you everything you need to know about the nutrients that enable your body to run in tip-top condition. Then, in Chapter 6, I help you adapt your diet to give you essential nutrients while avoiding reflux. Finally, Chapter 7 is a really interesting compilation of home remedies (including some foods) for heartburn. (For your amusement, I include some curiosities, such as an old-time herbal recipe for a heartburn cure, which is so yucky that when you read it, you'll see that this remedy is definitely something that you shouldn't try on your own!)

Part III: Treating Your Middle

Chapter 8 is a straightforward guide to finding and working with doctors for heartburn relief. Chapter 9 lists the tests that the doctor is likely to suggest to pinpoint the source of your tummy troubles. Chapter 10 is a catalog of heartburn medicines, and Chapter 11 gives you a catalog of drugs that can actually give you heartburn. Chapter 12 (snip, snip) explains surgical remedies for heartburn.

Part IV: Creating a Comfortable Lifestyle

Chapter 13 tells you how to make your body strong and supple, which certainly sounds nice, in relation to your quest to conquer heartburn. In Chapter 14, I talk about how to deal with unhealthy habits such as smoking. Chapter 15 lays out stratagems for avoiding stress. Chapter 16 tells you how to furnish your home and clothe your body without triggering heartburn.

Part V: Meeting the Special Cases

Heartburn isn't a one-size-fits-all condition. Some folks, in special circumstances, have special problems that require special solutions. Chapter 17 discusses the special risks and remedies for heartburn during pregnancy. Chapter 18 examines the littlest heartburn sufferers: infants and children. Chapter 19 approaches heartburn among the aging.

Part VI: The Part of Tens

In true *For Dummies* fashion, I get out my top-ten lists for this part. Chapter 20 debunks heartburn myths, some of which you may still believe are true. In Chapter 21, I provide a list of really reliable Web sites for people with digestive disorders. And Chapter 22 lists common digestive conditions you probably don't have — but should know about, just in case they pop up in your future. Or in the life of someone near and dear to you.

Icons Used in This Book

Icons are a useful *For Dummies* way to catch your attention and highlight information. They come in various shapes and forms.

When you see this guy, the accompanying text is solid, hands-on information that you can put to work.

This fabulous piece of art accompanies info that I don't want you to forget.

This icon alerts you to issues or occurrences that may prove harmful to your health or throw you a curveball in the battle against heartburn.

Though the info accompanying this icon is utterly fascinating, it's not necessarily critical to your understanding of the topic at hand. Feel free to skip it if you want.

Though you need to run all things health and heartburn related by your doctor, this icon reminds you when the waters are especially choppy or murky and a doctor's guidance is especially critical.

Where to Go from Here

One of the best things (among many) about a *For Dummies* book is that each chapter is a self-contained unit. You don't have to start at Chapter 1 and work through the rest of the book in order. And you don't have to read it cover to cover to benefit from the information. You can dive right in anywhere and be certain of finding everything you need to know about the subject at hand. Splash!

Part I
Naming Your Pain

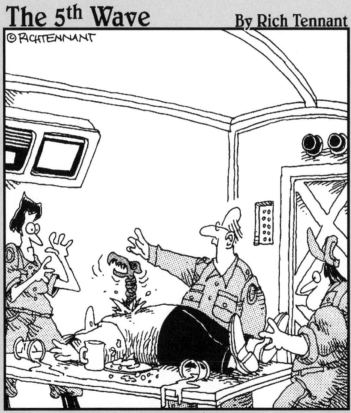

The 5th Wave   By Rich Tennant

"Relax everyone! It's _not_ heartburn, _not_ acid reflux, just an internal alien implantation!"

In this part . . .

To start healing the burn, you need to know the basic facts about heartburn, reflux, and gastroesophageal reflux disease, a real mouthful that's usually abbreviated as GERD. This part defines heartburn, explains the workings of your digestive tract, lists the symptoms and consequences, and tells you who's at risk.

Chapter 1

Picturing Heartburn and Reflux

In This Chapter

▶ Getting acquainted with heartburn, reflux, and GERD

▶ Understanding what puts the *burn* in heartburn

▶ Exploring treatment options

This chapter is Numero Uno for a very good reason: It serves as your introduction to heartburn, reflux, and the impressively tongue-twisting gastroesophageal reflux disease (GERD).

If you already know that heartburn, reflux, and GERD are common and painful but treatable, then you can just skip along to Chapter 2, which explains your entire digestive system, from one end to the other, with special emphasis on the parts involved in heartburn, reflux, and GERD.

But if you're not totally sure that you know what these conditions are, how they happen, and what tricks modern medical science has up its collective sleeve to alleviate your discomfort, then stick around for a couple of pages.

You can pick up some facts about heartburn's impact on your life, some new words to describe exactly what you mean when you say, "Gastroesophageal reflux disease," and some basic guidelines on what type of help is out there and where you can go to find it.

Meeting Your Heartburn

Do any of these situations sound familiar?

> ✔ Dinner was yummy. But now, just an hour later, you feel that burning pain in the lower part of your chest — and maybe have a nasty taste in your mouth.

- ✔ You're out for short run, pounding the pavement, when you round the corner and that burning pain makes another appearance.

- ✔ You lie down to sleep, and as you're about to drift off to Dreamland that pain pops back up, right smack in the middle of your chest.

If you didn't hurt so much, you'd probably see this saga as sort of boring and predictable: No matter what you do, no matter where you are, that sudden pain can bring you up short, halt the action, take the wind out of your sails . . . okay, I'm done with the metaphors.

The fact that you bought this book and are thumbing through Chapter 1 tells me that you've already met the pain that most of the world calls heartburn. Now, the time has come to get to know a little more about it.

Saying hello to your fellow sufferers

When you hurt, the natural reaction is to think that you're alone in your misery. But the first fact that you need to know about heartburn is that its pangs are as common as the common cold.

In fact, according to the National Institute of Diabetes and Digestive and Kidney Diseases (NIDDK) — I have no idea why that abbreviation doesn't read NIDDKD — the incidence of heartburn is positively staggering.

- ✔ More than 60 million American adults have heartburn at least once a month.

- ✔ More than one-third of American women ages 35 to 44 and slightly less than one-third of American men in the same age group have "frequent" heartburn. Translation: More than two incidents a week.

- ✔ At least 25 million Americans have heartburn every day.

- ✔ One in four pregnant women has heartburn daily; a lot of babies whose parents think they have colic actually have heartburn; and as you get older, your risk of heartburn rises — which explains why, later on in this book, you can find a chapter devoted to each of these three "special" groups (Chapters 17, 18, and 19, to be specific).

And don't think Americans have the market cornered when the discussion concerns heartburn:

- ✔ According to a study published in the medical journal *Gut,* up to 20 percent of the people in Great Britain have heartburn at least once a week.

✔ According to the *Canadian Medical Association Journal,* about

- 7 percent of all Canadians suffer from heartburn daily.

- 13 percent of all Canadians suffer from heartburn once a week.

- 24 percent of all Canadians suffer from heartburn at least once a month.

Quantifying your discomfort

According to a Gallup poll conducted for the American Gastroenterological Association (AGA), a professional organization for doctors who treat digestive disorders,

✔ More than 80 percent of people with heartburn say that their condition stops them from enjoying food.

✔ More than 60 percent of people with heartburn say that their pain keeps them from getting a good night's sleep.

✔ More than 40 percent of people with heartburn say that their pain interferes with their ability to concentrate at work.

✔ More than 30 percent of people with heartburn say that their pain gets in the way of enjoying family activities.

In other words, having heartburn is no fun at all. And it's not a matter to take lying down (especially right after you eat, a common invitation to heartburn). As the stats show, heartburn can really affect your quality of life. But you don't have to "just deal with it." Your doctor can help alleviate the discomfort (a topic that I cover in the "Looking for Help in All the Right Places" section later in the chapter).

Pinning the Tail on the Heartburn Donkey

Wine, hot dogs, chocolate, orange juice, hot pepper . . . Why go on? Chances are, you see this list of positively deee-li-cious foods as a red flag emblazoned with the words *Heartburn Ahead!* Ditto for smoking, working out, or being stressed. No surprise there.

The surprise is that although some lifestyle choices, such as avoiding certain foods, eating smaller meals, giving up cigarettes or alcohol, adjusting your exercise regimen, or trying to avoid stressful situations, may relieve your symptoms, heartburn isn't a lifestyle disease.

Actually, that point deserves to be mentioned again: *Heartburn isn't a lifestyle disease.* The pain in your middle is the most common symptom of an honest-to-goodness medical condition called *gastroesophageal reflux disease,* generally abbreviated as GERD.

Defining terms and conditions

Like most medical conditions, GERD has a vocabulary all its own. To be able to talk about heartburn, you need to know a few basic terms.

- **Esophagus:** This term comes from the Greek words for *to carry* and *to eat.* The *esophagus,* or the throat, is the approximately 8-inch tube that connects the back of your mouth (the *pharynx*) with your stomach.

- **Lower esophageal sphincter (LES):** The *LES* is a muscular valve between the esophagus and the stomach. When you swallow, the valve opens to let food into the stomach. Then it should close tightly enough to keep acidic stomach contents from flowing backwards into the esophagus.

Because you need to know how the LES works — and malfunctions — to understand heartburn and reflux, and because the *For Dummies* books are designed to let you jump in at any point, this book repeats the LES definition more than once. Feel free to skip it after you have it down pat.

- **Reflux:** Grammatically speaking, reflux is double-jointed, a word that can be either a noun or a verb. *Reflux,* the noun, is the acidic liquid that sloshes back through the LES into your esophagus. *Reflux,* the verb, is what happens when the LES malfunctions. So you can correctly say, "His LES opened by mistake, allowing reflux to reflux into his esophagus."

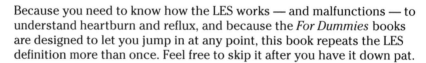

Talking Brit versus Yank

Americans and Britons speak the same basic language. But sometimes they pronounce the same word differently — in the United States, *schedule* is *skedule;* in Britain, it's *shedule.* And they often spell words differently, too. You go to the *theater* in New York, but the play's on stage at the *theatre* in London. Red's a *color* in Chicago, but hop over the Big Pond to Liverpool, and red's a *colour.* In Los Angeles, teachers expect to *civilize* their students; in Manchester, the plan is to *civilise* them.

Medical words aren't immune to these interesting variations. If you're reading this page in Canada, the United Kingdom, Australia, New Zealand, or any place else where your friends and neighbors speak British English rather than American English, *esophagus* starts with an *o.* In other words, *esophagus* becomes *oesophagus,* and *GERD* morphs into *GORD.* Who else would tell you these things?

✔ **Frequent reflux:** Everyone has an incident of reflux at least once in his life, but some people have reflux a lot more often. Doctors call reflux that occurs more than two or three times a week "frequent reflux."

✔ **Heartburn:** This is the sharp pain that you feel as soon as reflux flows through the LES to hit the lining of your esophagus.

No, heartburn has nothing to do with your heart. No, it isn't really a burn, as in you touched a lit match and singed your finger. But the sharp pain in the middle of your chest can feel like a burn, or sometimes like the searing pain of a heart attack. In fact, heartburn may so closely mimic the sensation of a heart attack that your doctor may actually have to run special tests to differentiate the two conditions (as Chapter 3 explains). So, heck, if it occurs in the region of your heart and it sometimes feels like a heart problem, why not call heartburn "heartburn"?

✔ **GERD:** GERD is an abbreviation for **g**astro**e**sophageal **r**eflux **d**isease, the most accurate term for the condition characterized by frequent reflux. Because fewer people have GERD than have occasional heartburn or occasional reflux, throughout this book you see the words *heartburn* and *reflux* much more often than you see *GERD*.

Pain isn't the only sign of reflux. You may also have bad breath, a dry cough, and several other symptoms that I describe in Chapter 3. If you're burning with the desire to find out whether your heartburn fits the pattern, bookmark this page and flip ahead to the symptoms checklist in Chapter 3. Then come back for an overview of the ways in which your doctor can help you put out the fire.

Looking for Help in All the Right Places

Sooner or later, as your heartburn continues to burn its way into your life, you will come to the following decision: I need help! Saying these words out loud (or even thinking them) makes you one smart cookie. Acting on them expands your smartness exponentially, a term mathematicians use when they mean "a whole bunch."

The National Heartburn Alliance (NHBA) is an organization dedicated to publicizing the effects of heartburn and finding ways to relieve your discomfort. Every few years, the alliance does a survey of Americans to find out what's what with heartburn and how they begin to look for help. One recent NHBA survey says that

- More than half the people with heartburn say that their pain makes it hard for them to enjoy life.

- 90 percent of the people with frequent heartburn tried to find relief with simple over-the-counter (OTC) remedies.

- Only 20 percent of heartburn sufferers have gone on to seek serious medical advice and relief.

What in the world is holding back the other 80 percent?

Modern medicine's cup brimmeth over with heartburn remedies, so your doctor will have treatment to ease your discomfort. (For more about the doctors who treat heartburn, see Chapters 8 and 9).

Editing the menu

What you eat, when your eat it, and how much you eat aren't the first causes of your reflux-related heartburn. But — and it's a big "but" — these activities can exacerbate your symptoms. As Chapter 6 explains, avoiding foods on your personal heartburn list, eating smaller portions, and never eating right before you lie down to sleep may all make you feel much, much better.

As you fine-tune your menu, avoiding some foods and emphasizing others, be careful to follow a healthful diet that provides all the vitamins, minerals, and nutrients a body needs. For more on how to do that, see Chapter 5.

Looking at your lifestyle

Like food choices, style choices didn't give you heartburn in the first place. But living smart can make you much more comfortable, and I provide you with the strategies to do just that in Chapters 13, 14, 15, and 16 — heck, make that the entire Part IV. For example, savvy fashionistas (and fashionistos) know that when you have GERD, your clothing can matter. Wearing clothes so tight that you have to lie down on the bed to zip them is a no-no because clothes that are tight around your middle put pressure on your stomach, pushing it up against your LES . . . . And take my word for it — this isn't a good thing. Ditto for smoking, abusing alcohol, and doing the "wrong" exercises.

Remedying the situation

Have heartburn only once in a while? Some of Granny's home remedies are effective enough for Granny's grandson, the doctor, to endorse them. One example is sodium bicarbonate, or baking soda. Read all about home remedies, including some you should avoid, in Chapter 7.

Managing your meds

A whole medicine cabinet awaits the heartburn sufferer, starting with simple antacids available over the counter, no questions asked, and progressing up the pharmaceutical ladder to prescription-strength products that reduce the amount of acid that your stomach pumps out naturally each day. Faced with this dazzling array of magical meds, you'd be smart to consult with your doctor, who's qualified to guide you through the maze. Before you go, though, check out Chapter 10 to arm yourself with a few basic facts on heartburn meds and Chapter 11 for medications that may make your heartburn worse.

Seeing the surgeon

For a relatively small number of people with heartburn, when no other treatment seems effective, some doctors may suggest heartburn surgery to alter the innards, tightening the LES. You can read about this procedure in Chapter 12, including the fact that some experts say this elective surgery is virtually never warranted.

Chapter 2

Tracking Your Digestive Tract

Digestion is a 24/7 operation built around the well-designed tube — narrow in some places, wide in others — that begins at your mouth, continues down through your throat to your stomach, and then winds on to your small and large intestine and through the colon to end at your anus.

With contributions from your liver, pancreas, and gallbladder, this digestive disassembly line processes every usable component of the foods you eat and the liquids you drink into simple compounds your body can burn for energy or use in building new tissue. Then, equally efficiently, your digestive system compresses the indigestible residue to be eliminated as waste.

Are you the kind of person who can't leave a nutritional molecule or fact unturned? Then you need a copy of my book *Nutrition For Dummies, 3rd Edition* (Wiley Publishing, Inc.), which has an exhaustingly detailed description of the digestive process.

This chapter is a shorter version. (If the folks behind the *CliffsNotes* brand published their take on digestion, it may look a lot like this.) It begins with a lickety-split tour of the digestive tract and then moves on to explain how some parts of your food-processing system may suddenly malfunction, triggering reflux, leading to heartburn.

So fasten your seat belts. To paraphrase Bette Davis in *All About Eve,* it's going to be a bumpy ride.

Defining Digestion

Digestion is the process of changing food into a form that the body can absorb and use as energy or as the raw materials to repair and build new tissue. It's a two-part process, half mechanical, half chemical.

- *Mechanical digestion* begins in your mouth as your teeth tear and grind food into small bits and pieces you can swallow without choking. The muscular walls of your esophagus, stomach, and intestines continue mechanical digestion, pushing the food along, churning and breaking it into smaller particles.

- *Chemical digestion* occurs at every point in the digestive system, beginning when you see or smell food. These sensory events set off nerve impulses from your eyes and nose that trigger the release of *enzymes* and other substances that will eventually break down food to release the nutrients inside. The body then burns these nutrients for energy or uses them to build new tissues and body parts.

Virtually every organ in your digestive system plays a part in both mechanical digestion and chemical digestion, so before I get to the nitty-gritty, check out the refresher in Table 2-1 on which body parts play a role in the process. (And check out Figure 2-1, which maps each of these players in the digestive game.) In the following sections, I outline the process from beginning to end.

Table 2-1	Mechanical and Chemical Digestion	
Organ(s)	*Mechanical Digestion*	*Chemical Digestion*
Eyes, nose, and brain	N/A	Send "alert" messages to digestive tract.
Mouth	Teeth break food into small pieces. Tongue pushes food to the back of the mouth and into the esophagus.	Saliva moistens and compacts food. Salivary enzymes begin to digest carbohydrates.
Esophagus (throat)	Esophageal muscles push food to stomach. Saliva lubricates throat.	N/A

Organ(s)	Mechanical Digestion	Chemical Digestion
Esophagus (throat)	The lower esophageal sphincter (LES), a trapdoor between esophagus and stomach, opens to allow food into the stomach; closes to prevent reflux.	
Stomach	Stomach muscles contract to break food into smaller particles, mashing food into a mass called *chyme.*	Stomach glands secrete stomach juices, including hydrochloric acid and specialized enzymes to digest protein and fat.
Small intestine	Intestinal muscles push food through the small intestine.	Digestive enzymes from the pancreas and bile from the gallbladder continue the process of breaking food into nutrients, which are then absorbed through intestinal walls and sent through the blood stream to other parts of body.
Large intestine	Muscle contractions compact waste to feces.	Resident bacteria digest amino acids from proteins.
Rectum/ anus	Muscle contractions push waste through the anus.	N/A

Demystifying *metabolism*

The process by which your body extracts nutrients from food and uses the nutrients as energy or building materials for tissues and chemicals such as enzymes is *metabolism,* from *metabole,* the Greek word for *change.*

The metabolic process that converts molecules of nutrients to energy is called *catabolism,* from *katabole,* the Greek word for *casting down.*

The metabolic process that uses molecules of nutrients to build new tissues is called *anabolism,* from *anabole,* the Greek word for *a rising up.*

Boy, the guy who first said, "It's all Greek to me," sure hit the nail on the head.

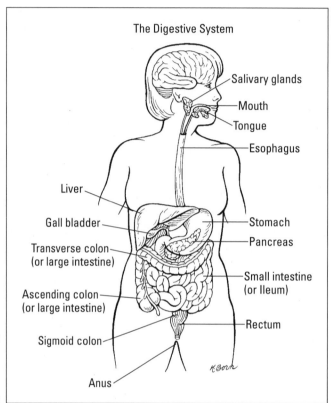

The Digestive System

Salivary glands

Mouth

Tongue

Esophagus

Liver

Gall bladder

Stomach

Pancreas

Transverse colon
(or large intestine)

Small intestine
(or Ileum)

Ascending colon
(or large intestine)

Rectum

Sigmoid colon

Anus

Figure 2-1:
Diagramm-
ing digestion.

Seeing and smelling

At first glance — or sniff — the link between your eyes, nose, and stomach sounds a tad weird. But think about it: How many times has the sight or scent of something yummy like a simmering stew or baking bread set your tummy rumbling?

The sight of an appetizing dish or the aroma (actually scent molecules bouncing against the nasal tissues) sends signals to your brain: "Good stuff on the way." As a result, your brain — the quintessential message center — shoots out impulses that

✔ Make your mouth water.

✔ Make your stomach contract (hunger pangs).

✔ Make intestinal glands start leaking digestive chemicals.

All that from a little look and sniff. Imagine what happens when you actually take a bite!

Tasting and chewing

You know that small bag of potato chips you have stashed way at the back of your desk drawer? Well, dig it out and take a chip.

After all, this is *Heartburn & Reflux For Dummies,* not *Dieting For Dummies,* by Jane Kirby, R.D., (Wiley) so you have my permission to forget about any diets you may be pondering for a minute to put that chip right smack into your mouth. (Need I mention that if you can't stop at one chip, or ten, or 100, you may want to pick up a copy of *Dieting For Dummies?* Or my book *Weight Loss Kit For Dummies?* Nah.) So bite into that chip.

As the chip hits your tongue, your mouth acts as though someone had thrown the "on" switch in a fun house.

- ✔ Your teeth chew, breaking the chip into small manageable pieces.

- ✔ Your salivary glands release a watery liquid (*saliva*) to compact the chip into a mushy bundle (a *bolus* in digestive-geek speak) that can slide easily down your throat on a stream of saliva.

- ✔ *Enzymes* (which you can think of as digestive catalysts in this case) in the saliva begin to digest carbohydrates in the chip.

- ✔ Your tongue lifts to push the whole ball of wax . . . no, bolus, back toward the *pharynx,* the opening from your mouth to your esophagus, and then through a muscular valve called the *upper esophageal sphincter,* which opens to allow the food through. In other words, you're about to swallow.

Swallowing

I call it the *esophagus.* You call it the *throat.* To-may-to, to-mah-to . . . either way when I talk about swallowing, I'm talking about sending food down the approximately 8-inch tube that connects your mouth to your stomach.

As food enters the esophagus, your salivary glands release a rush of saliva to help food slide more easily down the tube. Then your esophageal muscles swing into action.

Like the rest of your digestive tract, your esophagus is ringed with muscles that contract to produce wavelike motions — which you can refer to as *peristalsis* or (no surprise here) *peristaltic contractions,* if you're so inclined — pushing food down toward your stomach.

At the bottom of the esophagus — an area known as the *gastroesophageal junction* — a muscular valve called the *lower esophageal sphincter* (LES) opens to allow food through. Then the LES closes to prevent *reflux,* the flow of stomach contents back into the esophagus. A malfunctioning LES is public enemy No. 1 in the reflux world.

If you're familiar with your digestive system's functions, but want to know more about the LES, right now, this minute, what the heck! Indulge yourself. Skip ahead in this chapter to the section "Examining the LES."

Mixing and mashing

Point to your stomach. Go ahead. Don't be shy. Odds are your finger is aimed somewhere around your belly button, an interesting site to be sure, but definitely not your stomach. Your stomach, a wide, pouchy part of the digestive tube, is located on the left side of your body above your waist and behind your ribs.

Like the walls of your esophagus, the walls of your stomach are strong and muscular. They contract with enough force to break food into ever smaller pieces as glands in the stomach walls release *stomach juices* — a highly technical term for a highly acidic blend of enzymes, hydrochloric acid (HCl), and mucus. The stomach juices begin the digestion of proteins and fats into their respective bodily building blocks — amino acids and fatty acids.

Churned by the stomach walls and degraded by the stomach juices, what started as food — apples, pears, potato chips, steak, cake, you name it — is now a thick, soupy mass called *chyme* (from *chymos,* the Greek word for *juice*). The stomach's wavelike contractions push this messy but still intact substance along to the small intestine where your body begins to pull out the nutrients it needs.

Extracting the good stuff

If you didn't quite pass the point-to-your-stomach test in the previous section, don't worry. You can pick up some participation points here with an easy anatomy lesson.

Open your hand and put it flat slightly below your belly button, with your thumb pointing up and your pinky pointing down. Your hand is now covering most of the relatively small space into which your 20-foot-long small intestine is neatly coiled. (Don't ask me who bought the naming rights to this organ. Twenty feet doesn't seem that small to me either.)

Waste management through the ages

Digestion involves waste. Producing waste is one thing. Getting rid of it is something else, like a problem that has plagued man- and womankind for centuries. Historians know that several early civilizations, including the ancient Romans, built systems to bring water into the city and carry waste away, and Charles Panati, author of *Extraordinary Origins of Everyday Things* (Perennial) says members of the Minoan royal household enjoyed the first-ever flush toilet more than 4,000 years ago.

The Chinese are also reputed to have built a flush toilet, but in most of the world, the commode of choice for several thousand years was the chamber pot, a waste container stored under a bed or inside a cabinet and emptied out the window — sometimes onto passersby.

The first modern Western flush toilet was the "water closet," also known as the WC, built for Britain's Queen Elizabeth by her godson John Harrington in 1596. The kid had fallen from royal favor for passing around "racy Italian fiction" so he was looking for a way to make up. She liked the *loo* (Brit-talk for "toilet"), but Harrington earned her ire once again by writing a book about his invention.

The next advance in flush toilets arrived in 1775. Harrington's toilet had washed waste into a box where the stuff sat and stank. British math whiz Alexander Cumming took a great leap forward by curving the waste pipe on his toilet backward and putting a trapdoor between waste and bowl. A mere 100 years later, Cumming's stink-free toilet was standard bathroom furniture in Great Britain (Queen Victoria had a toilet decorated with gold, as well as the first ceramic toilet) and in the United States, thus setting the stage for the next advance in bathroom products: toilet paper.

The Brits beat the Americans to the flush toilet, but the colonists won the war on toilet paper. According to Joseph Nathan Kane's classic tome, *Famous First Facts* (H.W. Wilson), the first bathroom tissue was the "unbleached pearl-colored pure manila hemp paper" sold by New Yorker Joseph C. Gayetty at 5 cents for 500 sheets. Twenty-two years later, the Scott Brothers, Edward and Clarence of Philadelphia, packaged their paper as rolls, thus ensuring their fortune and the future of modern waste management.

Just like your esophagus and stomach, contracting muscles line your small intestines to push food along.

But your small intestine is nobody's copycat. This part of your digestive system has its own set of digestive juices including

- ✔ Alkaline goop from the pancreas that powers special enzymes (called *amylases*) to digest carbs

- ✔ Bile from the liver and gallbladder that acts as an *emulsifier* (a compound that enables fats to mix with water)

- ✔ Pancreatic and intestinal enzymes that complete the separation of proteins into amino acids

More contractions shove the chyme along the intestines while specialized cells in the intestinal walls grab onto sugars, amino acids, fatty acids, vitamins, and minerals, which are then sent off into your body for energy or as building blocks for new tissue.

Then, after your small intestine has squeezed every last little bit of useful material (other than water) out of the food, the indigestible remainder (think dietary fiber) moves toward its inevitable end in your large intestine.

Creating compost

Your large intestine is also sometimes called the colon. Think of this area as a giant sponge and press whose only jobs are to absorb water from the mass you deliver to it and then squeeze the dry leftovers into compact bundles of waste — which you may know as feces and your 2-year-old brother, nephew, son, or grandson may call poo-poo.

After resident colonies of friendly bacteria digest any amino acids remaining in the waste and excrete smelly nitrogen — in a process scientists call *passing gas* — muscular contractions in the rectum push the feces out of your body, and digestion's done.

Testing the Protectors

Your digestive system has three safeguards designed specifically to protect you from the burning sensation — heartburn — you experience if stomach contents accidentally slip back into your esophagus.

The word *reflux* describes the flow of acidic stomach contents back into your esophagus. The term used to describe the back-flow of actual food into your esophagus is *regurgitation.* And, if the regurgitated material comes all the way up into — and then out of — your mouth, you're *vomiting.*

These three digestive protectors are

- **Your esophageal muscles:** If stomach contents slide back up into your esophagus, your muscular esophageal walls contract involuntary, creating waves that push food back down into the stomach where it belongs.

- **Your lower esophageal sphincter:** Ladies and gentleman, may I introduce (or reintroduce, as the case may be) to you the famous (sometimes infamous) LES. The LES is your first and primary line of digestive defense, charged with keeping stomach acids and food in your stomach where they belong.

✔ **Your salivary glands:** You know that your salivary glands release saliva to help food slide into and down your esophagus. These helpful glands also release extra saliva to neutralize small amounts of gastric acids that may back all the way up into your esophagus. You can think of the salivary glands as the last line of defense against acid reflux. Problem solved.

Your salivary glands and your esophageal muscles are important in protecting you against reflux and regurgitation. Chapters 3 notes some medical conditions that may interfere with the ability of these two supporting players to counter reflux and lay out the list of people who are at risk of heartburn due to these failures.

But, the remainder of this chapter focuses on the undisputed star of the reflux drama — the LES. You can't understand heartburn and reflux without knowing how the LES is supposed to function, and what happens when things go awry.

Examining the LES

Your body contains plenty of circular parts such as your eye's pupil and many tubular parts such as

✔ Blood vessels

✔ Components of the respiratory tract such as the *trachea* (windpipe)

✔ Ducts carrying secretions from glands (such as the pancreas) into organs

✔ Parts of the urinary tract such as the *ureters* (the tubes through which urine flows from the kidney to the bladder) and the *urethra* (the tube through which urine flows out from the bladder)

✔ Sections of the reproductive tract such as the *fallopian tubes* (through which eggs move from the ovary to the uterus) and the vagina in women, and the *epididymides* (the tubes that transport sperm) in men

✔ Segments of the digestive tract, such as the esophagus and the intestines

Without some way to close all these tubes, material would flow in and out without any control. The device Mother Nature came up with was the sphincter. In medical-speak, a *sphincter* is a ring of muscles encircling the opening of a tube or circular organ such as the ones listed in the previous bulleted list.

The sphincter, which features most prominently in this book, is, of course, the lower esophageal sphincter or LES, the ring of muscles at the place where the esophagus meets the stomach (see Figure 2-2).

Important though it may be to your digestive comfort, the LES isn't your body's only important sphincter. Table 2-2 lists some others. After you skim the list, I move on to the LES.

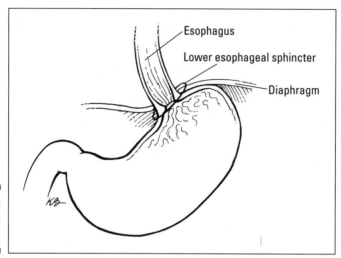

Figure 2-2:
Locating
the LES.

Table 2-2	Lords of the Ring Muscles
Sphincter	*Where It Is*
Boyden's sphincter	Between the gallbladder and the small intestine
External anal sphincter	At the outer opening of the rectum
Pyloric sphincter	At the opening between the stomach and the small intestine
Sphincter pupilae	Surrounding the eye's pupil
Sphincter urethrae	At the urethra's opening
Sphincter vaginae	At the vagina's external opening

Closing the door: Reviewing the life and times of the LES

Most of the time your LES remains tightly closed, sealing off the connection between the stomach and esophagus. What keeps the LES closed? Good question. The LES is made up of a special type of muscle. Most muscle is loose, or not contracted, when it's just sitting around. The LES muscle (and muscle from many other sphincters) is different. The LES muscle is normally contracted (a tight LES) and only relaxes with swallowing.

When you start to swallow, everything changes. As food moves from your mouth to your esophagus,

1. The upper esophageal sphincter at the back of your mouth opens.

2. The LES relaxes, opening the pathway to the stomach to prepare for the arrival of the food.

3. The muscle in the esophagus contracts and pushes the food down to and through the open LES.

4. After the food you're swallowing slips past your LES, the pressure picture reverts to normal and your LES closes so that the food doesn't slip back up.

Operating out-of-bounds

As a rule, the food you put in your mouth goes down your esophagus, and then — gulp! — through the LES into your stomach. You don't even have to think about these actions because the LES opens automatically as you swallow food and then shuts tight again to prevent food from slipping back.

Was that a belch? Or a burp?

Neither. According to *Stedman's Medical Dictionary,* the correct term is *eructation,* "the voiding of gas or a small quantity of acid fluid from the stomach through the mouth."

✔ Eructation comes from *eructare,* the Latin root for the activity called *belching.*

✔ Belch can be traced to the Anglo-Saxon word *bealcian,* meaning *to bring up, emit, splutter out.*

✔ Burp is a slightly softer modern American/English synonym first heard around the 1920s. As a noun, burp describes the sound you make when you belch. As a verb, burp describes what you do to help an infant belch up air, usually after eating.

The definition of belch and burp are standard English, but both belch and burp also have secondary meanings as slang terms. You can probably fill in your own list!

For example, some dictionaries of slang terms say that belch may be a complaint or (when applied to a human being) a drunken derelict. As for burp, the slangsters point to its adoption as an adjective used to describe the fast noisy machine pistol — the burp-gun — used by the Germans during World War II and a second weapon, a submachine gun used by the Russians during WWII and for some time after.

Frequent fliers have their own slang use for burp. You know that neat paper bag with the fold-in plastic seals in the seat pocket in front of you on an airplane? One obvious name for the bag is — you got it! — the burp bag, sometimes also called a "barf bag." By the way, "barf" is a college term for upchucking, which is pretty slangy on its own.

But some determined people can open the LES at will. Remember when you were 8 or 9 years old and hard at work discovering how to belch? Okay, you would never, ever have done anything that gross, but you probably knew other people who did. The point is that the trick you (yeah, yeah, I know; those other rude kids) discovered how to perform was to swallow air and relax the LES so that stomach gas could erupt in a glorious belch.

The LES may also open spontaneously at other times when you're not swallowing food or trying to belch. These spontaneous LES openings, called *transient LES relaxations,* are most common

- ✔ When your stomach is full after eating
- ✔ When you have swallowed air, which may happen when you're breathing rapidly, when you're nervous or excited, or when you've had a swig of a bubbly carbonated drink

Transient LES relaxations can be useful. A belch enables you to expel excess air from your stomach, relieving a sensation of bloat. The downside of transient LES relaxations is that the belching may also allow some food and stomach juices to slosh back into your esophagus.

If reflux occurs as the result of transient LES relaxations, the involuntary esophageal contractions that I mention earlier in the chapter (in the "Testing the Protectors" section) push the reflux material back down into your stomach where it belongs. At the same time, your salivary glands release a rush of extra saliva to neutralize any acid in your esophagus.

In a normal, healthy digestive system, the reflux caused by transient LES relaxations is minor, and these measures are sufficient to prevent heartburn.

Suffering with a good muscle gone bad

Everyone experiences transient LES relaxations, but people with GERD experience the problem more frequently than other people do. In addition, people with GERD may have natural pressure on the LES, producing a sluggish sphincter that simply refuses to stay.

This kind of LES misbehavior leads to reflux not only after eating or while belching but also when

- ✔ Bending over
- ✔ Lying down
- ✔ Sleeping
- ✔ Wearing tight clothes

The acid test

Question: What is pH? **Answer:** My freshman chemistry book defines pH as "the negative logarithm of the H_3O concentration."

Q: Say what? **A:** Sorry. Plain English: pH is a number that describes the acidity of a water-based solution such as household ammonia, black coffee — or even your stomach's gastric juices.

Q: Who invented pH? **A:** Søren Peter Lauritz Sørensen, a Danish biochemist at the Carlsberg Laboratory in Copenhagen, created the pH system in 1909.

Q: What do the letters *pH* stand for? **A:** Sorenson's system equates acidity with the presence of hydrogen particles called hydronium ions (the artists formerly known as hydrogen ions), so he chose the term pH for *pondus hydrogenii* (Latin for *potential hydrogen*) as his measure. The higher the concentration of hydronium ions, the more strongly acid the solution. The lower the concentration of hydronium ions, the less acid the solution. Both very strong acids such as HCl and very strong bases such as lye have one thing in common: both are extremely corrosive.

Q: What's acid and what's not? **A:** The pH scale ranges from 0 to 14 (some solutions do score higher or lower). Acids are grouped at the low end. For example, a solution of HCl — the acid your stomach releases to dissolve food — is a 1, meaning it is a very strong acid. Lemon juice is a 2. That cola in the glass next to your computer is a 3.

Q: What's the opposite of an acid? **A:** A base, formerly known as an alkali. Basic (alkaline) solutions score at the higher end of the pH scale. For example, oven cleaner is a 14.

Q: How does pH figure in my body? **A:** I thought you'd never ask. Your body is very sensitive to pH changes. Even a slight variation may interfere with a normal chemical process such as the exchange of impulses between nerve cells or the manufacture of compounds such as enzymes.

If the pH of the liquids in a certain area rises or falls, your body rushes to neutralize the offender and restore the proper balance. One relevant example is the salivary glands' releasing saliva to neutralize stomach acids flowing back into your esophagus. When your own body can't do the job, you may need to call in a support team such as antacids products to do the job.

Here's the pH of some common solutions.

1 HCl (very acidic)
2 Stomach juices
3 Beer, soft drinks
4 Tomato juice
5 Black coffee
6 Urine

7 Water, human blood
8 to 9 Seawater
10 Milk of magnesia
11 Household bleach
13 to 14 Drain cleaner (very basic)

The result is a continuous back-flow of acidic stomach contents into the esophagus, triggering the burning sensation called heartburn and raising the risk of other problems associated with damage to the esophagus's lining. (For more on the symptoms and consequences of GERD, check out Chapter 3.)

 All this talk of acids backing up from the stomach to the esophagus may raise a few questions. Why does the same acidic gastric juice that is so valuable as an essential aide to digesting food in your stomach become a problem if it splashes into your esophagus? Basically, Mother Nature designed the lining of your stomach to tolerate stomach acids; the lining of the esophagus isn't as acid-resistant.

Tall cells called *columnar epithelium* line the inside of your stomach. These cells are columnlike — meaning tall, not flat. Columnar cells link up to form an acid-resistant layer of stomach lining called the *columnar mucosa.* The lining of the esophagus, on the other hand, is made up of flat cells called *squamous epithelium* (by the way, *squamous* means flat). The *squamous mucosa* is a layer of flat cells that are much more sensitive than the columnar mucosa to stomach acid.

Even very short exposure to stomach acids may damage the squamous mucosa lining the esophagus, but the columnar mucosa lining the stomach just laughs at daily acid baths, mainly because it is able to secrete a substance (mucus) that neutralizes the acid before it causes damage. The subject of this book isn't ulcers, but I'll throw this nugget in anyway: When that mucus is damaged (maybe by a bacteria or some medications), then the good old columnar mucosa breaks down and you get stomach ulcers.

Chapter 3

Cataloging the Symptoms and Hazards of Heartburn, Reflux, and GERD

In This Chapter

▶ Listing the symptoms of gastroesophageal reflux disease (GERD)

▶ Considering the complications and consequences of GERD

*Y*our throat is tight; you have a cough. Is it the flu — or is it gastro-esophageal reflux disease (GERD)? You're wheezing, and you've got a postnasal drip. Is it an allergy — or is it GERD? You have a pain right smack in the middle of your chest. Is it a heart attack — or is it GERD?

GERD is one of nature's great mimics, with symptoms so similar to the symptoms of other common medical conditions that you often can't tell the players without a scorecard. Does that mean you can never, ever be sure that what you have is GERD? Absolutely not. The point of this chapter is to enable you to sort through your symptoms and unmask the great pretender. Then, in the words of the great Sherlock Holmes: "When you have eliminated the impossible, whatever remains, *however improbable,* must be the truth." Or to put it another way: If it walks like a duck, and talks like a duck, then duck! It's GERD.

In this chapter, I describe the primary symptoms of GERD, including heartburn and reflux, in order to help you identify the source of that annoying pain in your middle. Next comes a guide to the possible complications of constant reflux. After reading this part, you can understand why you need to discuss your symptoms with your doctor.

Tracking the Symptoms

As you can read in practically every chapter in this book, the most important player in the heartburn-reflux-GERD drama is your lower esophageal sphincter, often identified simply by its initials, LES. The LES is a valve located at the point where the esophagus meets the stomach. When you swallow, the valve opens to permit food to enter the stomach. Afterwards, it's supposed to shut tight to prevent *reflux* — acidic stomach contents — from flowing backwards, or *refluxing,* into your esophagus.

A malfunctioning LES may open accidentally. The subsequent reflux produces an entire catalog of unpleasant reactions, each a recognized symptom of GERD. In the following sections, I explicitly explain each symptom for your enlightenment, starting at the top, your mouth.

Monitoring your mouth

When acidic stomach contents reflux back into your esophagus, your salivary glands react instinctively, secreting *saliva,* a natural antacid, in an attempt to neutralize acids in your esophagus and stomach. The result of reflux in this area of your body may be

- **Bad breath:** A bad taste isn't the only thing reflux leaves in your mouth. You may also experience the really unpleasant smell of regurgitated stomach stuff.

- **Water brash:** This term describes a flood of excess saliva and acidic liquids rising from your esophagus into your mouth. Some experts say this thick, whitish liquid looks like beaten egg whites, but its pleasant appearance is belied by its taste: nasty and bitter.

Bringing up baby

Infants who experience the GERD symptoms listed in this chapter don't yet know the words to tell you how bad they feel. Identifying infant reflux requires your sharp, observant eye. Watch for a baby who

- Fails to gain weight

- Hiccups often

- Is hoarse or has a persistent cough

- Is irritable for no clear reason

- Often chokes on food

- Seems hungry but refuses to eat

Report these symptoms to your pediatrician. If your bundle of joy has GERD, the doctor can offer help. You can also read up on the unique challenges of infant and childhood reflux in Chapter 18.

By neutralizing acid, simple over-the-counter (OTC) heartburn products such as the antacids listed in Chapter 10 may temporarily alleviate the bitter taste and possibly stinky smell of reflux. Some people with occasional reflux may find that plain breath mints or chewing gum is a simple way to counter the taste and smell.

As with all reflux symptoms, you need to rule out other possible causes. In this case, you want to ensure that dental problems (such as an infection) aren't at fault before attributing the bad taste and bad smell to GERD.

Exploring your respiratory tract

Time out for a quick anatomy lesson. When you swallow or take a breath, the food you eat or the air you breathe starts off down the same path. But then it comes to a fork in the road at the *pharynx,* the opening at the back of your mouth. Your pharynx branches into the two separate tubes:

- ✔ **Your esophagus:** This tube carries food to your stomach.
- ✔ **Your trachea:** Also, known as your *windpipe,* this tube carries air to your lungs.

Everything sounds nice and neat to this point. But the entrance to your esophagus is really close to the entrance to the trachea. A piece of food or sip of liquid meant to go into the esophagus might accidentally go into the trachea, an uncomfortable situation accurately described as "going down the wrong pipe." Now think about this happening in reverse.

When acidic liquids splash back from your stomach through your LES into your esophagus, they may just bounce all the way up to the pharynx and then crossover to spill down into the trachea. If this mishap occurs once in a while, then it's no big deal. But frequent crossover reflux may lead to well-known warning signs of GERD:

- ✔ Chronic cough
- ✔ Frequent throat clearing
- ✔ Sore throat

Ah, but there's more. When reflux runs down your trachea to your *larynx,* also know as your *voice box,* you may experience

- ✔ Chronic laryngitis
- ✔ Hoarseness
- ✔ Wheezing

These three signs of GERD are most likely to occur if you suffer from night-time reflux, a situation more accurately labeled *sleep-time reflux.* Why is sleeping conducive to reflux? Because, when you lie relatively flat on your back, your stomach is above your esophagus (as I explain in Chapter 16). As a result, acidic stomach contents flow more easily through a lazy LES to your esophagus and on to your pharynx where they may follow a path of least resistance to your trachea.

Changing your sleeping position is one way to reduce your risk of nighttime reflux. A second possibility is to avoid lying down with a full stomach, which might press up against your LES. And skip your customary midnight milk and cookies (as I suggest in Chapter 6). You can have them tomorrow.

Examining the esophagus

The esophagus is GERD's main staging area, site of its most classic symptom: *heartburn* — a sharp, burning sensation right in the center of your upper abdomen caused by acid reflux hitting the delicate esophageal tissues.

Heartburn due to reflux is so common that you may assume that anyone with reflux has it. On the contrary, as the National Institute of Diabetes and Digestive and Kidney Diseases (NIDDK) points out:

- ✔ Everyone with GERD has reflux.

- ✔ Not everyone with reflux has heartburn.

- ✔ But anyone who has heartburn more than twice a week should be evaluated for GERD.

Describing heartburn's burn

Heartburn really hurts. The pain is in the middle of your chest, but it may also radiate out to your neck and shoulder. Sometimes the discomfort may be severe enough to mimic the pain of one of two forms of heart disease, angina or *myocardial infarction,* the medical term for a "heart attack."

- ✔ **Angina:** A pain in the center of your chest caused by a temporary decrease in the flow of oxygenated blood to your heart muscle.

- ✔ **Heart attack:** Characterized by pain that begins in the center of your chest and may radiate to your neck, shoulder, and left arm. The pain is caused by a blockage in an artery preventing the flow of oxygenated blood to the heart.

Separating heartburn from heart disease

Sometimes, the pangs of severe heartburn may be so difficult to differentiate from those of a heart attack that your doctor may haul in the really sophisticated equipment such as an EKG (electrocardiogram) to check for an irregular heartbeat, which points to angina, or blood tests to look for the presence of enzymes related to heart damage. Other times, your doctor may want to do exercise stress tests or even a *cardiac catheterization* (a test where dye is injected into your heart to look for blockages) prior to declaring that the problem isn't your heart.

More often, however, he simply evaluates the symptoms to make a *differential diagnosis,* the medical term for the process used to decide which condition a set of symptoms fits. Table 3-1 lists some of the factors doctors consider to distinguish the pain of heartburn from the pain of heart disease.

Table 3-1	Is It Heartburn? Or Is It . . .?
Condition	**Pain Characteristics**
Angina	Usually triggered by exercise
	Usually relieved by rest
Heart attack	Intense and prolonged, not relieved by home remedies such as antacid
	Radiates to neck and jaw
	Radiates to upper arms (especially the left arm)
	Accompanied by sensation of pressure on the chest *plus* feelings of lightheadedness, nausea or heavy sweating, shortness of breath, or all these symptoms, all at once
Heartburn	Usually follows a meal
	May be related to position (for example, bending or lying down)
	Sharp, but usually relieved quickly with antacids

Warning! Heart attack in progress!

Sometimes a pain in the chest really is a *heart attack*. The longer the heart and brain are deprived of oxygen-toting blood, the worse the damage will be. Clearly, the faster a heart attack victim gets medical attention, the better his or her chances of surviving with minimal injury.

As soon as you suspect that someone (maybe you) is having a heart attack, the American Heart Association (AHA) recommends taking (or giving) one 325-milligram aspirin. Aspirin is a blood-thinner; the AHA says taking it at the onset of symptoms may lower the risk of dying by 23 percent.

Next, don't panic, but do move quickly. Dial 911 or the Emergency Medical Service to summon an ambulance staffed by EMS technicians trained to treat heart-attack victims. The ambulance is likely to get to you faster than you can get to the hospital, especially if you're the one having the heart attack and would have to drive yourself.

If you know how to perform CPR — the abbreviation for *cardiopulmonary resuscitation*, a technique that can provide vital oxygen for someone having a heart attack — this is the time to put your skill to work. If not, put this book down right now, and call your local chapter of the AHA or the address of the nearest class. Or log on the AHA site (www.americanheart.org), and find the CPR link. You can find a CPR class near your home by entering state and zip code. It's worth repeating: Learn CPR and you may save someone's life.

Checking your personal list of symptoms

The moment of truth has arrived. You have that pain in the middle of your chest. Again. Is it GERD? Only your doctor can say for sure. If you mark the "yes" box more than once on Table 3-2, the smart money says, "Ask him." You have nothing to lose but that fire in your chest.

Table 3-2	Do I Have GERD?		
Sign		*Yes*	*No*
I often have bad-tasting foam in my mouth.		❑	❑
I often have bad breath (even though I have no dental problems).		❑	❑
I clear my throat several times a day.		❑	❑
I cough a lot.		❑	❑
I am frequently hoarse.		❑	❑
I often have laryngitis.		❑	❑
I wheeze (even though I don't have asthma).		❑	❑
I have heartburn more than twice a week.		❑	❑

Calculating Long-Term Consequences

The really good news is that most people with heartburn or reflux can lead normal, happy lives after they get their GERD under control by:

- ✔ Watching what — and when — they eat (see Chapter 6)
- ✔ Altering their lifestyle to avoid heartburn triggers such as cigarettes (see Chapter 14)
- ✔ Choosing effective medication (see Chapters 10 and 11)

The not-so-hot news is that some people simply ignore their heartburn. By doing this, they're making a serious mistake. Left untreated, GERD's continuing reflux of acidic stomach contents into the esophagus may trigger a cascade of complications such as those listed by the NIDDK:

- ✔ **Inflammation of the esophagus,** leading to
- ✔ **Esophageal ulcers and bleeding,** leading to
- ✔ **Esophageal scarring,** leading to
- ✔ **Esophageal *stricture* (a narrowing of the tube) or damaged muscles,** leading to
- ✔ **Difficulty in swallowing** or to
- ✔ **Precancerous changes in the esophageal lining,** leading to
- ✔ **Esophageal cancer**

Not a pretty picture. But — back to the good news — with expert assistance, you can short-circuit the progression and protect your delicate esophagus from heartburn.

Irritating the environment

Remember when you were a kid and you skinned your knee and your mom poured on some antiseptic? Remember the burn, the redness, and the misery of it all? Acid reflux does exactly the same thing to your esophageal lining that the pavement and the antiseptic did to your knee.

When reflux hits, it reddens and inflames the mucous membrane lining your esophagus making it sting like all-get-out. After that, repeated inflammation may wear away the esophageal lining, producing *esophageal erosion* (esophageal *ulcers*). Splashing more reflux on the ulcers can trigger bleeding.

Stop! Esophageal bleeding is a genuine red flag that says, "Get this body to the ER. Stat!" (Medical shorthand for, right now, this minute, what in the world are you waiting for?)

Some people have symptoms of reflux but no signs of inflammation, a condition some people call *non-erosive esophageal reflux disease* (NERD). People with NERD — no, this isn't a joke — may also experience the characteristic sting of heartburn, perhaps from injury to nerves just beneath the surface of the esophageal lining.

Swallowing hard

Meanwhile, the injured esophageal lining fights back by producing new cells that form tissues called *scars.* Repeated scarring may thicken the esophageal lining, creating *esophageal stricture,* a narrowing of the tube that makes pushing food down to your stomach difficult.

The reflux-related muscle damage may also affect your ability to swallow. As Chapter 2 explains, your digestive tract is essentially one long tube with muscular walls that contract in movements called *peristalsis,* shoving food along from your mouth to your anus. Damaged muscles don't contract as effectively. This interruption of the peristaltic movements stops food dead in its tracks, wherever it happens to be. If it happens to be in your esophagus, you may feel a choking sensation.

Changing cells: Barrett's esophagus risk

Tissues injured by reflux make repairs by producing new cells to form scars. But when healthy cells are injured again and again, they may just give up and metamorphose into different, less-healthy cells, a condition called *metaplasia. Squamous cells* (the type of cell usually found in the esophagus) are replaced with *columnar cells* (the type of cell usually found in the stomach and intestines). Depending on whose stats you choose to use, anywhere from 9 to 15 percent of the people with long-term reflux undergo this cellular surrender and conversion. The end result is a condition called *Barrett's esophagus.*

Strangely enough, people with Barrett's esophagus often feel less reflux-related pain because the new metaplastic tissue is less sensitive than normal mucous membrane. The catch: Pain is the body's warning signal. People who don't feel pain don't look for relief. As a result, their reflux-related esophageal damage continues unabated and metaplastic cells enter a new, precancerous phase called *dysplasia.* Dysplasia is totally silent.

But silent doesn't mean safe. According to the Society of Thoracic Surgeons (guys who operate on the chest), for people with Barrett's esophagus, the risk of developing esophageal cancer is 30 to 125 times higher than for people who don't experience reflux. Which brings me to the most serious potential consequence of untreated gastroesophageal reflux disease: Esophageal cancer, which deserves all the respect you can give it.

Before I tackle that issue, check out these two online sources for more info on Barrett's esophagus:

> ✔ **The Cleveland Clinic, Center for Barrett's Esophagus:** `www.cleveland clinic.org/gastro/barretts`

> ✔ **Johns Hopkins University, Barrett's Esophagus page:** `http://pathology2.jhu.edu/beweb`

Facing the facts about esophageal cancer

Heartburn is common. Esophageal cancer isn't. According to the American Cancer Society, less than 1 percent (0.4 percent to 0.5 percent) of the people with Barrett's esophagus progress to esophageal cancer in a given year. The lifetime risk is related to how many years you live with the condition, but most experts say that a Barrett's patient's risk of getting cancer in his or her lifetime is less than 5 percent.

There are actually two types of esophageal cancer. One is a complication of long-term acid reflux (*adenocarcinoma*), and the other probably isn't related to reflux, but is related to excess use of tobacco and alcohol (*squamous cancer*). Adenocarcinoma is more common in the United States. Squamous cancer is more common in other parts of the world (for example, the incidence in northern China, India, and southern Africa). As Table 3-3 demonstrates, the number of cases of both kinds of esophageal cancer and, sadly, the number of deaths, have been rising steadily in the United States over the past 30 years.

Table 3-3	Esophageal Cancer in the United States	
Year	*New Cases*	*Deaths*
1973	5,500	6,488
1980	8,020	7,985
1990	10,380	9,719
2000	11,770	12,232
2004	14,250 (estimate)	13,300 (estimate)

Source: *American Cancer Society*

Identifying people at risk

- **Men:** The National Cancer Institute says both types of esophageal cancer are three to five times more common among men than among women.

- **African Americans:** Squamous cell esophageal cancer is three times more common among American black men than among American white men. NCI says African American women are also at higher risk than Hispanic and non-Hispanic white women.

- **Middle-aged and senior citizens:** Both types of esophageal cancer are most common among people ages 45 to 70.

- **Smokers and drinkers:** Both alcohol and tobacco smoke irritate the esophagus, but neither one alone is as potent a risk factor as the two together. Why? Scientists theorize that alcohol acts as a solvent for carcinogens in burning tobacco, carrying them into the esophageal lining. This may be more of an issue in squamous cell esophageal cancer, but it's likely true in both types.

- **People who eat their food very hot:** Foods and beverages consumed very hot irritate the esophagus; theoretically they may raise the risk of repeated injury leading to cell changes leading (mainly) to squamous cell cancer.

Predicting outcomes and drawing conclusions

Esophageal cancer isn't a walk in the park. Forty years ago, only 1 to 4 percent of Americans diagnosed with this disease lived for at least five years. Today, while the five-year survival rate has risen to 9 to 13 percent, and many patients live much longer, this cancer is still highly lethal.

Having said all this, I'm going to draw some practical conclusions. First, don't ignore your symptoms. Second, don't ignore your symptoms. Third, don't ignore your symptoms. Treating GERD successfully is easier than treating Barrett's esophagus, which is easier than treating esophageal cancer. Got the picture? Good.

Chapter 4

Rating Your Reflux Risk

In This Chapter

▶ Drawing a picture of heartburn

▶ Defining your family ties to heartburn

▶ Tying in gender

▶ Listing medical risks

▶ Explaining why weight matters

▶ Determining your own risk

*W*ho gets heartburn? Are you at risk? This straightforward chapter answers these two basic questions. But wait; there's more: You get a definition of risk factors, a list of what's risky, advice on how to take the bite (and the burn) out of some risky conditions, and last but not least a questionnaire that enables you to assess your chances of ending up at the antacid counter (or in your doctor's office) sooner or later.

Picturing People with Heartburn

Who has heartburn? Men? Women? Old people? Young people? People who live in cities? People who live on a farm? Healthy people? Sick people? Tall people, short people, thin people, overweight people? All kinds of people?

In the spring of 2003, the National Heartburn Alliance (NHBA) conducted the latest in its series of nationwide surveys designed to answer these *burning* questions (and anyone with heartburn knows that's exactly the right adjective). What they found was: Everybody gets heartburn. You can check the study out for yourself at www.heartburnalliance.org. Just click the link to the NHBA survey results.

Defining the terms

The easiest way to estimate your chances of getting heartburn is to add up your *risk factors* — the single traits or events statistically linked to an increased risk of — well, anything, but most commonly illness and death. For example, eating high-fat foods is a risk factor for reflux. So is smoking. So don't eat fatty foods, don't smoke, and you'll avoid heartburn, right? The absolutely, totally definite answer is . . . maybe.

The truth: The link between risk factors and risk is strictly statistical. For example, when researchers such as the ones who ran the NHBA survey collect information about people with reflux, they find that reflux is more common among smokers and eaters feasting on fat. The catch is that not every smoker or everyone who eats lots of high-fat foods has reflux. In other words, eating high-fat food and smoking are risk factors that make it *more likely* but *don't guarantee* that you'll develop reflux.

Classifying reflux risk factors

As a general rule, the risk factors for heartburn and reflux fit neatly into one of three basic categories:

- ✔ **Risk factors you can't change:** Reflux seems to run in families, and the associated risk factors are often issues you can't do anything about.

- ✔ **Risk factors whose effects you can lessen but not entirely eliminate:** Your health and medical history may present risk factors (such as diabetes) whose riskiness you can reduce but not eliminate simply by getting (and following) good medical advice and treatment.

- ✔ **Risk factors you can eliminate:** This category is home to lifestyle choices that include heartburn-risky behavior. You can take charge and change these bad habits: Change your diet, be more (or less) active, toss the ciggies, and so on.

What? You're still smoking? You haven't read Chapter 14 yet? You haven't checked out *Quitting Smoking For Dummies* by David Brizer, MD (Wiley)? What are you waiting on?

Table 4-1 groups broad heartburn risk factors into these three basic categories. When you finish this chapter, you'll be able to take steps to reduce some of your risk factors.

Yes, your weight is listed in two categories. Why? Because to a larger (ouch!) extent, your body size and shape are a product of your genes, but what you eat also obviously affects your possibility of picking up *excess* weight. *Ipso facto* — Latin for "it's a fact" — weight weighs in, in two categories.

Table 4-1	Reflux Risk Factors	
Risk Factors You Can't Change		
Gender		
Weight (body shape/size)		
Family history		
Risk Factors You Can Make Less Risky		
Certain illnesses and medical conditions		
Food allergies/sensitivities		
Certain necessary medicines		
Risk Factors You Can Eliminate		
Irritating foods and beverages		
Meal schedule/meal size		
Weight (obesity)		
Lifestyle (exercise, smoking, living conditions, emotional stress)		

Factoring In the Family

Does your mom have heartburn? Is your dad a reflux-er? Do six of your cousins and your great-aunt Jane head for the antacids after dinner? If you were born into a heartburn clan, your risk of suffering from the ailment is probably higher than average. If nobody related to you has reflux, lucky you! But your family ties — like your gender (see the next section) — are a risk factor you can't change. The reasons are boringly clear. Your genes influence

- ✔ **Your body type:** Human beings sometimes resemble pieces of fruit. People with apple-type bodies are round around the middle; people who look like pears are broad around the bottom. Being a member of an apple-shape family (and having an apple-shape body yourself) is a risk factor for heartburn.

- ✔ **The structure of your body parts:** The lower esophageal sphincter (LES) is the trapdoor between your esophagus and stomach, Ordinarily, the LES closes tight after you swallow food. A loose LES may open accidentally to allow acidic stomach contents back into the esophagus. The result? Heartburn. Not surprisingly, a floppy LES may run in families. Score two risk factors.

✓ **Your risk of certain chronic conditions:** "Mentioning Medical Risks," later in this chapter, is an entire section listing medical problems that may raise your risk of reflux. For the moment, just consider that some of these conditions, such as asthma and diabetes, tend to run in families. Score three.

Do three strikes mean you're out in the heartburn game? To use a phrase you find repeatedly in books about medicine and medical conditions, *not necessarily.*

Your family history may put you at risk, but you don't just have to sit there and take it. Being forewarned — remember Mom, Dad, those cousins, and your great-aunt Jane? — you know it's smart to check with your doctor if you begin to experience the same kind of digestive discomfort. So what are you waiting for?

Big town, big burn? Not necessarily

During the National Heartburn Alliance's 2003 heartburn study, NHBA researchers questioned more than 5,000 people from sea to shining sea in search of the city, town, or village where Americans are most affected by heartburn/reflux. The questions were part of a "Burn Factor Index" — the NHBA's way of assessing heartburn's effects on a person's life. For example, the NHBA wanted to know: Does heartburn interfere with your social life? Does heartburn keep you from work? Does heartburn prevent you from getting a good night's sleep? How often do you use antacids? How often do you use prescription products?

In the end, when the scientists toted up the scores, 24 U.S. cities came out on top. No, the winners (losers?) weren't the stressful big cities like New York City and Los Angeles. In fact, smaller cities seem to be the worst places for a heartburn sufferer to call home.

Right now, nobody knows why. One possibility is that Big Town folk are normally so overstressed that they consider heartburn a minor annoyance, and therefore didn't report their heartburn to researchers, while smaller towners are seriously annoyed when something like heartburn plays heck with their normally mellow lives. While you're waiting for the next study to explain it all, take a look at the 24 U.S. cities that scored highest in heartburn complaints among responders to the *NHBA 2003 National Survey.*

1. Charlotte, NC	13. Milwaukee, WI
2. Jacksonville, FL	14. Pittsburgh, PA
3. Roanoke, VA	15. Boston, MA
4. Louisville, KY	16. Raleigh, NC
5. Denver, CO	17. Baltimore, MO
6. Spokane, WA	18. Albany, NY
7. Miami, FL	19. Salt Lake City, UT
8. Tampa-St. Petersburg, FL	20. Columbus, OH
9. Atlanta, GA	21. Cincinnati, OH
10. Grand Rapids, MI	22. Omaha, NE
11. Orlando, FL	23. Des Moines, IA
12. Minneapolis-St. Paul, MN	24. Peoria, IL

Rendering a Gender Bias

Women are more likely than men to have heartburn. Why? Hormones. And more hormones. In fact, a woman's hormones affect her risk of reflux most directly at two specific points in her life: during pregnancy and after menopause.

Expecting trouble

When she's pregnant, a woman secretes extra amounts of the two female hormones, *estrogen* and *progesterone*. Both are natural muscle relaxants that enable the uterus's muscular walls to expand to make room for the fetus, which is good. The problem is that these hormones also relax

- ✔ The muscular walls of the esophagus so that they no longer push food as efficiently down into the stomach
- ✔ The muscular LES, which no longer snaps shut as tightly as it should
- ✔ The stomach's muscular walls, which no longer push food as efficiently out of the stomach and into the small intestine

Result? Food moves more slowly down the esophagus, you have a loose LES, and your full stomach pushes up against the LES. In other words, you have the perfect preamble to, yes, reflux. (For more about coping with pregnancy-related risks of reflux, check out Chapter 17.)

Linking estrogen to heartburn

In 2002, scientists at the Karolinska Institute in Stockholm released the results of two surveys after the institute studied more than 60,000 Norwegians and gathered tons of data on who gets reflux and why.

A no-risk surprise

After you know that your family history, your gender, and your body size and shape are risk factors for reflux, you may think that your age also belongs on the list. Well, yes — and no. Although older people are more likely than younger people to have heartburn, reflux may actually pop up at any time from infancy (see Chapter 18) to older age (see Chapter 19). In other words, age may be a risk factor. Or it may not. What can I say? Life is a puzzle.

The Swedes discovered that heartburn is significantly higher before menopause than after *unless an older woman chooses to use hormones.* According to the Swedes' Norwegian data:

✔ Using hormone replacement therapy (HRT) (estrogen plus progestin) produces a risk of reflux slightly higher than the risk for women who don't use hormones.

✔ Using estrogen alone doubles the risk.

✔ Using estrogen alone and being obese (body mass index higher than 35; see Chapter 13 for more on BMI) produces a risk 33 times higher than that for nonobese women who don't use hormones (see the "Weighing Weight's Weight on Reflux" section later in the chapter for more on weight as an independent risk factor).

The explanation? Both hormones and excess weight loosen the LES.

Mentioning Medical Risks

As I explain in-depth in Chapter 2, reflux is what happens when your LES, the trapdoor between the esophagus and stomach, opens to allow stomach contents back into the esophagus. Moreover, several common medical conditions weaken the LES and increase your risk of reflux. If you have one of the conditions on this list, sorry, you're at higher risk. Ladies and gents: The envelope, please.

Asthma and other respiratory problems

The frequent coughing and straining to exhale common among people who have asthma may cause your stomach or your abdominal muscles to press against the LES.

Seasonal allergies or a simple (sorry, miserable) common cold and cough may trigger the same symptoms and lead to a temporary round of reflux-related heartburn.

Diabetes

You probably didn't know that one complication of diabetes is a slowdown in the time it takes for food to move out of your stomach on its way into the small intestine. Why does this matter? Because the longer food lingers in your stomach, the greater the possibility that your full stomach will press up against the LES, nudging it open and raising the risk of reflux.

If you have frequent heartburn, eating smaller meals may reduce the risk of reflux — whether or not you also have diabetes (check out Chapter 6 for more mealtime advice).

Hiatal hernia

Your *diaphragm* is the muscle that stretches across the inside of your torso, separating your abdomen (which houses your stomach and intestines) from your chest. The place where the esophagus goes through the diaphragm is called the *hiatus*. Sometimes the following can put extra pressure on your diaphragm, causing it to pull away from the esophagus:

✔ Coughing

✔ Sudden physical exertion

✔ Vomiting

✔ Obesity

✔ Pregnancy

The result is a *hiatal hernia*. Check out Figure 4-1.

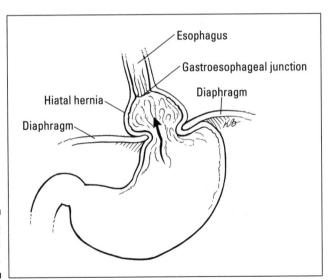

Figure 4-1:
The gap in
the wrap.

Small hiatal hernias are common, especially as people grow older. Interestingly enough, most people with hiatal hernias never know they have them. Things change, however, if the part of your stomach pushing up through the gap in your diaphragm nudges your LES open, permitting stomach liquids to reflux into your esophagus. Even then, however, your doctor may not have to treat the hiatal hernia directly because

- ✔ Antireflux medicines usually relieve your heartburn (see Chapter 10).
- ✔ The only treatment for a hiatal hernia is surgery (see Chapter 12).

Scleroderma

The literal definition of *scleroderma* — from the Greek words *sclero-* (hard) and *derma* (skin) — is *hardening of the skin.* People suffering from scleroderma develop skin that looks as though it has hardened. The hardened appearance is caused by an overproduction of connective tissue called *collagen* under the skin, which stretches and tightens the skin above.

Scleroderma may also thicken and swell muscle tissue, such as the muscles lining the digestive tract. As a result, food doesn't move along smoothly from your esophagus to your stomach and on through the intestines, thus increasing the risk of reflux.

Scleroderma is an *autoimmune disease,* a condition in which the body reacts to its own tissues, in this case connective tissue. Other autoimmune diseases such as systemic lupus erythematosus, also known as SLE or lupus, and rheumatoid arthritis, may also affect the esophageal muscles, but rarely as seriously as scleroderma.

Zollinger-Ellison syndrome

With this rare condition, a small tumor produces a hormone (*gastrin*), which causes the body to make too much acid. If your reflux is particularly difficult to control or is associated with ulcer disease or perhaps diarrhea, your doctor may check the level of gastrin. If your gastrin is really high, your doctor may need to order more tests to make sure you don't have Zollinger-Ellison.

Weighing Weight's Weight on Reflux

If you've read my book *Controlling Cholesterol For Dummies* (Wiley), you may recognize this heading. I like it so much, that I decided to use it again. Years and years of scientific studies and surveys show that excess poundage produces a higher risk of *morbidity,* the scientific term for illness, and *mortality,* the scientific word for you-know-what. You don't know what? Okay: I can spell it out — d-e-a-t-h.

Table 4-2 shows some of these problems caused by being seriously overweight. Notice something missing from the list? Right: Reflux. Not to worry. In this section, I define obesity and explain how it affects your risk of reflux.

Table 4-2	Weight-Related Health Conditions
Condition	*Weight Connection*
Gallstones	Overweight and/or rapid weight loss leads to the formation of gallstones.
Gout*	Obese people often have high blood levels of *urates,* irritating byproducts of protein digestion linked to attacks of gout.
Incontinence	Excess weight weakens pelvic muscles, leading to urine leakage.
Osteoarthritis	Excess weight stresses joints.
Sleep apnea	Excess weight weakens muscles at the back of the throat that hold the airway open, causing you to stop breathing — and wake up — for a few seconds as many as hundreds of times a night.

*A form of arthritis that occurs primarily (9 to 1) in men

Counting extra pounds

The totally modern way to weight your weight is the Body Mass Index (BMI), a measurement introduced in 1990 by the National Heart, Lung, and Blood Institute.

BMI is a unisex measure of weight relative to height, a number — such as 24 — that serves as a predictor of your risk for weight-related illnesses such as diabetes, high blood pressure, heart disease, stroke, gallbladder disease, and arthritic pain. The higher your number, the higher your risk. In a nutshell, here's how to calculate your BMI:

1. **Divide your weight in pounds by your height in inches squared.**

2. **Multiply the result of Step 1 by 705.**

I provide examples and tons of additional information on BMI and weight control in Chapter 13. For now, just recognize that, based on health statistics and death rates provided by the National Institutes of Health (NIH), a whole bunch of experts from the American Heart Association (AHA) to the American Dietetic Association and the American Society of Bariatric Physicians (doctors who deal with weight issues) agree with the following:

✔ BMI lower than 18.5 is *underweight.*

✔ BMI of 18.5 to 24.9 is *healthy weight.*

✔ BMI of 25 to 29.9 is *overweight.*

✔ BMI of 30 is *obese.* (***Note:*** Some studies mark obesity at BMI 35.)

✔ BMI over 40 is *extremely obese.*

Linking weight and reflux

The bottom line: Your bottom line matters, especially if you're an apple-shape person whose bottom line is the middle of your body.

Theoretically, toting extra pounds around your middle increases your risk of heartburn because

✔ Abdominal fat press up against your stomach.

✔ Your stomach presses up against your LES.

✔ Your LES opens, allowing acid stomach contents back into your esophagus.

The *Karolinska* study that links estrogen or hormone replacement therapy to a higher risk of reflux (see the "Linking estrogen to heartburn" section earlier in this chapter) said "ditto" for a higher BMI.

✔ The average BMI for people with reflux in the *Karolinska* study was 28.1.

✔ Compared with men of normal weight (BMI between 18.5 and 24.9), the risk of reflux was 3.3 times higher for *Karolinska* men whose BMI is 35 or more.

✔ Compared with women of normal weight, the risk of reflux was 6.3 times higher for *Karolinska* women whose BMI is 35 or more. (BMI is gender neutral, so the normal weight for women in also between 18.5 and 24.9.)

This study makes the clear point that losing weight definitely can control your reflux, right? Ah, if only it were so.

Consulting contradicting evidence

Despite an apparently logical cause-and-effect relationship between obesity and reflux, the annoying fact is that some studies show that many people with heartburn continue to experience reflux even after they lose weight, sometimes even after they lose lots of weight.

But even if losing weight doesn't chase away your heartburn, controlling the poundage may help you feel better and reduce your risk of other medical problems, such as heart disease, high blood pressure, and diabetes. And that's as good as it gets in this imperfect world.

Pinpointing Problem Eaters

Stop. Before you read another word, put down this book, and go get yourself a pad and pencil or some sticky notes you can use as bookmarks. Paper clips, preferably the pretty pastel ones, are also useful.

This section requires you to switch back and forth among several different chapters, which is hard to do just by holding your finger in the section you've just left. You can use the pad and pencil to write down the pages to check and then check 'em all later, or you can place the sticky notes here, there, and everywhere for cross-reference. Or you can use those paper clips, or . . . well, you get the idea.

People whose lifestyle choices produce heartburn can change their behavior so as to make themselves more comfortable. No office supplies are required — just a bit of common sense and a serious dose of willpower.

Fatalistic foodies

These people eat anything on their plate even though they know that some foods and beverages such as alcohol, coffee, tea, carbonated beverages, and hot stuff (in the spicy sense; think red peppers and curry) are obvious trouble-makers. They figure that *everything* gives them heartburn, so why rule out a food that tastes good?

Wrong, wrong, wrong. As Abe Lincoln once said, "You may fool all the people some of the time; you can even fool some of the people all the time, but you can't fool all of the people all of the time." If he were talking about heartburn, old Abe may have changed that a bit to read:

✔ Some foods cause heartburn for some people some of the time.

✔ Some foods cause heartburn for some people all the time.

✔ But no foods cause heartburn for all the people all the time.

In other words, a smart person like you can edit her menu to avoid the worst offenders. Just turn to Chapter 6, which has neat charts from the NHBA rating the heartburn potential of practically every food you'll ever encounter and some suggestions on creating a heartburn diary to track the particular foods that burn you up.

Fast Eddies

Nobody knows for sure whether Beaver Cleaver's older brother's best friend wolfed down his food, but if he did, he was swallowing air right along with his burgers and fries.

Swallowing air isn't good. The air hangs around the LES, waiting for you to burp it up. When you do, your LES opens and guess what? Reflux.

Big eaters

Teenage boys seem to eat huge meals without any trouble, but that's not always true for everyone else. Large meals stretch the stomach, which pulls on the LES and increases reflux. Also, eating huge meals often makes you heavier — another risk factor for reflux. Just try eating smaller meals. If you feel better, you have your answer.

Anytime eaters

As Chapter 13 explains, eating right before a workout is a recipe for reflux. Ditto (Chapter 14) for eating right before you hop into bed. So don't do it. Ever.

Adding Up Your Own Reflux Risk

Now the time has come to estimate your very own personal risk of reflux. Why *estimate* rather than make an *absolute prediction?* Because the best thing about being human is that in this whole, wide world, you're the one and only totally unique you.

Regardless of the statistics and studies, when it comes to risk factors for heartburn (and everything else, too), your body may beg to differ. For example, coffee, especially the deep, rich, dark-roasted brews such as espresso, is a well-known heartburn trigger. But you may be the one person in a thousand, maybe even the one in a million, for whom coffee (including espresso) never, ever causes reflux.

And that brings me to the questions in Table 4-3. Look at each question and answer yes or no. If you already have heartburn, scoring lots of "yes" answers is a gentle way of saying you need to alter your behavior. If you have a few "yes" answers and don't yet have heartburn, you now have an idea of what's risky for the future. Take the hint to have an intimate chat with your doctor to make sure your risk stays as low as possible. No "yes" answers? You must be doing something right — including having picked the right parents.

Table 4-3	Adding Up Your Risks		
		Yes	*No*
I have lots of relatives with reflux.		❏	❏
I'm a woman.		❏	❏
I'm pregnant.		❏	❏
I'm past menopause.		❏	❏
I'm taking estrogen.		❏	❏
I have an apple-shape body.		❏	❏
My BMI is 30 or above.		❏	❏
I have asthma.		❏	❏
I have allergies that make me cough a lot.		❏	❏
I have diabetes.		❏	❏
I have a hiatal hernia.		❏	❏
I have taken antibiotics for an ulcer.		❏	❏
I'm a smoker.		❏	❏
I eat three large meals a day.		❏	❏
I eat very quickly.		❏	❏

Part II
Eating Your Way to Relief

The 5th Wave   By Rich Tennant

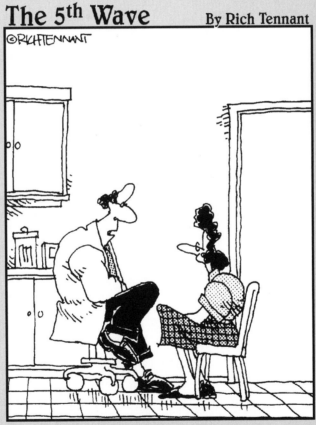

"A burning sensation in your chest can be a sign of reflux. The fact that the symptom only occurs when the pool boy is working in your backyard, however, raises some questions."

In this part . . .

When food triggers heartburn, you need expert advice on how to tailor your diet to get the nutrients you need. This part tells you all about the good stuff in food and then lays out a regimen for assembling a nutritious, delicious pain-free menu. It also delivers the scoop on herbal remedies and home grown cures — the good and the bad.

Chapter 5

Meeting Your Nutrition Needs

. . . .

. . . .

Sometimes people with reflux must avoid foods considered nutritional superstars. One good example is orange juice — a terrific source of vitamin C. Alas, some reflux patients say OJ makes them uncomfortable, which means they must hunt for other good sources of C. Strawberries come quickly to mind — just as long as strawberries don't trigger reflux. The same problem hits people who get gas from greens (thus missing heart-healthy folate) or milk (bone-building calcium) or, well . . . any number of good foods.

The list seems endless but the principle is clear: Tailoring your diet to your reflux may make getting all the nutrients you need more difficult. But, before you can figure out *how* to get the nutrients you need, you need to have a clear picture of exactly *what* nutrients you need. This chapter — which is a bit loooooong, but really important — lays out the list of nutrients considered essential for a healthy diet.

After you have this info under your belt, you can move to Chapter 6, which presents the pros and cons of specific foods for people with reflux. Together, these two chapters can make creating healthful menus that are kind to your digestive tract easier.

Measuring Nutrition

A healthful diet provides sufficient amounts of all the nutrients your body needs. The question is, how much is enough? The folks in charge of answering that question are the experts on the Food and Nutrition Board at the National Academy of Medicine, a division of the National Academy of Sciences. This distinguished group of nutrition gurus gets to decide every couple of years who needs how much of each nutrient in a balanced diet.

In 1995, the Board introduced the *dietary reference intake* (DRI), an umbrella term covering four different measurements for vitamins, minerals, and other good stuff.

- ✔ **Estimated average requirement (EAR):** The amount of a nutrient that meets the needs for half the people in a specific group such as teenage girls or men and women older than 70. Nutrition pros use EAR to judge whether the normal diet for a whole population, such as Americans, provides adequate amounts of essential nutrients (such as vitamin A, for example).

- ✔ **Recommended dietary allowance (RDA):** Introduced in 1941, the RDA is a recommended average daily intake of a nutrient that's large enough to prevent (but not cure) a deficiency.

  The nice thing about the RDA is that you can satisfy its requirements by averaging your nutrient consumption over several days. For example, the RDA for vitamin C for women is 75 mg. Eight ounces of fresh orange juice has 124 mg C, so you can have one glass on Monday, skip Tuesday, have a second glass on Wednesday and still meet your RDA for Monday, Tuesday, *and* Wednesday. (124 mg vitamin C × 2 days = 248 mg ÷ 75 mg [the RDA] = 3.3 days.)

- ✔ **Adequate intake (AI):** AI is a recommendation for nutrients that are considered important to your health but haven't yet been assigned an RDA. The nutrients currently in this category are the vitamins biotin and pantothenic acid and the minerals chromium, copper, fluoride, manganese, and molybdenum. You'll be pleased to know that new research info can bump an AI up to an RDA. For example, in 2001, choline got its RDA. Huzzah for choline!

- ✔ **Tolerable upper intake level (UL):** This measurement is the largest amount of a nutrient you can consume each day without risking an adverse effect. For example, the RDA for vitamin C for adult men is 90 mg; the UL is 2,000 mg, an amount that may cause an upset stomach and increase your risk of kidney stones. (In the "Setting limits" section later in the chapter, I provide a rundown on the upper intake levels for vitamins and minerals.)

Wait! I'm not finished. I have a few more terms for you. Dip into the nearest nutrition textbook, and you're likely to bump up against the terms *macronutrients* and *micronutrients*. The words translate respectively to "big nutrients" and "little nutrients," meaning that a healthy diet provides a lot more of the first group (protein, fats, and carbohydrates) than of the second (vitamins and minerals).

How much is a lot more? A whole lot. The DRIs for protein, fat, and carbohydrates, also known as *macronutrients* (macro = large), are measured in grams (g). Most vitamins and minerals, also known as *micronutrients* (micro = small), are measured in milligrams (mg) and micrograms (mcg). A milligram is ⅟₁₀₀ of a gram; a microgram is ⅟₁₀₀ of a milligram.

And I'm still not finished.

Vitamins A and E are special cases.

- ✔ Your body gets vitamin A either as *retinol* (preformed vitamin A) from animal foods, such as liver, or from *carotenes,* plant compounds you can convert to retinol. Thus the modern measurement for vitamin A is retinol equivalents (RE). One RE equals one microgram of preformed vitamin A. ***Caution:*** Some nutrition tables and vitamin supplement labels still list vitamin A in International Units (IU), another term used for counting amounts of vitamin D.

- ✔ You get vitamin E from *tocopherols* and *tocotrienols,* two classes of compounds found in plants. The most active of these compounds is alpha-tocopherols. Although many supplement labels list vitamin E in IU, the modern measurement is milligrams of alpha-tocopherols equivalents: mg per TE.

If all this nutrition terminology has made your head ache, sit back and relax with a DD (delicious dish) of something good to eat. No, DD isn't a bona fide nutrition term. I confess: I made it up. And now I'm done with this section.

Beginning with the Big Guys

Protein, fats, and carbohydrates — together, this trio of macronutrients represents most of the solid material in your food.

- ✔ Say hello to protein, and right away you know you're shaking hands with something special because protein comes from *proteios,* the Greek word for *prime.*

- ✔ Fats are one big, happy family whose chemical name — lipids — comes from *lipos,* the Greek word for *fat.* By the way, liquid fats are called oils; solid fats are called fat.

- ✔ Carbohydrates are etymological commoners, named for their components: carbon (*carbo-*) and water (*hydra-*).

Pumping protein

Proteins are construction workers, used to build, maintain, and repair cells and tissues. Dietary proteins are also essential for synthesizing other, specialized proteins in your body such as *enzymes* (compounds that help you digest foods) and *neurotransmitters* (compounds that enable you to send messages between nerve cells to power the physical reactions of your organs and system, everything from motion to vision to the transport of oxygen). Most wondrous of all, proteins build *DNA* and *RNA,* the compounds in every single body cell that carry your *genetic code,* the information that makes you a unique and special individual.

Table 5-1 is a list of some of the important specialized proteins in your body.

Table 5-1	Some Special Proteins	
Protein	*Found In*	*Job*
DNA/RNA	Cell nucleus	Transmits genetic code
Enzymes	Throughout the body	Facilitate biochemical reactions
Hemoglobin	Red blood cells	Carries oxygen
Lipoprotein	Blood plasma	Carries cholesterol
Myoglobin	Muscle	Carries oxygen
Myosin	Muscle	Forms muscle fibers

Your best dietary sources of high-quality proteins are foods from animals. Certain combinations of plant foods, such as rice and beans, also provide valuable proteins. (For more on combining foods to produce high-quality proteins, check out my book *Nutrition For Dummies* [Wiley].)

How much protein does a healthy body need? The current RDAs for protein are

- **Infants:** 2.0 grams protein for each kilogram (2.2 pounds) of body weight
- **Adolescents:** 1.2 grams for each kilogram (2.2 pounds) of body weight
- **Adults:** 0.8 grams protein for each kilogram (2.2 pounds) body weight

Facing the fat facts

With the exception of cholesterol (which has no nutritional value), fats are high in calories. Although fats suffer from an often-deserved bad reputation, they fill a number of essential roles:

- Your body uses fats to manufacture biochemicals, such as hormones, the digestive juice *bile* (check it out in Chapter 2), and fat-soluble vitamin D, which I discuss in the "Investigating Vitamins" section later in the chapter.

- You store fats as *adipose* (fatty) tissue in female breasts, hips, thighs, buttocks, and belly, or male abdomen and shoulders. These fat deposits shape your body, cushion your skin, insulate you from cold weather, and serve as emergency sources of energy.

✔ And for more of what you can't see. Inside your body, fatty tissues and cells wrap a protective layer around your organs, sheathe your nerve cells, strengthen your cell walls, and fill up your brain, which is mostly fat and cholesterol.

The most abundant sources of dietary fat are foods from animals or vegetable fats and oils.

There is no RDA for total fat other than the recommendation to keep fat intake to 30 percent or less of your total calories. Take these additional steps:

✔ Reduce your consumption of *saturated fat* (found primarily in foods from animals) and *trans fats* (chemically altered unsaturated fats that behave like saturated fats).

✔ Increase your consumption of *polyunsaturated fats,* the fats found primarily in plant foods.

For more on how to monitor your fats, check out *Heart Disease For Dummies,* by James R. Rippe, MD, (Wiley), and *Controlling Cholesterol For Dummies,* by myself and Martin W. Graf (Wiley).

Counting on carbohydrates

Carbohydrates are the start-your-engines nutrient, the primary source of *glucose,* the molecule your cells burn for energy. Yes, you can burn fats and proteins for energy, the premise of the Atkins diet. But burning protein and fat is much less efficient than pulling glucose out of carbs because, as anyone who has tried the Atkins regimen well knows, a high-protein/high fat meal plan produces a major loss of water. In other words, you pee a lot!

On the other hand, a carbohydrate-based diet also protects your muscles, which is why it's sometimes called a "protein sparing diet." This is how it works. When you need energy, your body looks for carbs first. If none are available — for example, because you're on a severe reducing diet or have a medical condition that prevents you from using the carbohydrates you consume or are starving — your body pragmatically begins to burn its own protein tissues (muscles). If this protein burning goes on long enough, you will run out of fuel and die. It's called starving to death.

Carbohydrates also

✔ Regulate the amount of sugar circulating in your blood, thus keeping your energy level on the level.

✔ Feed friendly bacteria in your intestinal tract that help digest food. (See Chapter 2 for more.)

✔ Help your body absorb calcium.

Pinching an inch: Calories versus pounds

What weighs more, the riddle asks, a pound of feathers or a pound of gold? The answer is simple: neither because "a pound is a pound, the world around." But how about this one? What weighs more on your hips: an ounce of dietary fat or an ounce of protein or carbohydrates?

When you're counting calories, the answer is an ounce of dietary fat. Ounce for ounce — actually gram for gram — proteins and carbs "weigh" less than fats. To be specific:

- One gram dietary fat = 9 calories
- One gram cholesterol = 0 calories
- One gram protein = 4 calories
- One gram carbohydrates = 4 calories
- One gram dietary fiber = 0 calories

Your best source of dietary carbohydrates is plant foods. Why? Because there are no carbs in foods from animals.

How many grams of carbohydrates do you need? The USDA food guide pyramid suggests that 45 to 60 percent of your total calories should come from carbs. One gram of carbohydrates has four calories. If you consume 2,000 calories a day, your carb allotment can be 225 to 300 grams a day (45 percent of 2,000 calories equals 900 calories; 900 calories divided by 4 equals 225 grams carbohydrates; 60 percent of 2,000 calories equals 1,200 calories; 1,200 calories divided by 4 equals 300 grams carbohydrates).

The RDA for the indigestible carb we call dietary fiber is currently 25 grams for a woman and 38 grams for a man.

Investigating Vitamins

Vitamins are organic chemicals, compounds that contain carbon, hydrogen, and oxygen. They occur naturally in plants and animals (including you).

Nutritionists group vitamins into two broad categories:

- **Fat-soluble vitamins:** These vitamins dissolve in fat, so you store excesses in your fatty tissue.
- **Water-soluble vitamins:** These vitamins dissolve in water, so you get rid of excesses in your urine.

These two definitions raise issues that we talk about in the sidebar "Sizing up the megadose mystery," later in this chapter. For now, consider how your body uses each of the following vitamins. I give you descriptions of a number of vitamins in the sections that follow, and you may want to check out the "Crunching the numbers" section later in this chapter for detailed tables showing the RDA for all these vitamins (and minerals, too).

Fat-soluble vitamins

The fat-soluble vitamins are A, D, E, and K. You can find the first three in all kinds of foods; you get the fourth form from food — or your very own intestinal tract.

Vitamin A

Vitamin A is the vision vitamin, a building block of a protein (11-cis retinol, if you're curious) in your *rods* (cells in the back of your eye that make it possible for you to see, even when the lights are low). Vitamin A also moisturizes your skin and *mucous membranes* (the slick tissue lining eyes, nose, mouth, throat, vagina, and rectum), keeping them smooth and supple. Finally, vitamin A promotes the growth of healthy bones and teeth, keeps your reproductive system in working order, and encourages your immune system to churn out the cells that you need to fight off infection.

The best source of preformed vitamin A is liver, which, alas, also has a lot of fat and cholesterol. Good sources of *carotenes* (plant compounds that your body can convert to vitamin A) are bright yellow and deep green fruits and veggies, such as cantaloupe, carrots, spinach, and kale.

Don't try to get your carotenes from pills. These supplements, popular a few years back, have been linked to a higher risk of some forms of cancer.

Vitamin D

Think "bones-'n-teeth nutrients," and you naturally think of calcium. But you should also be thinking "D" because without D, your body can't absorb the calcium that it requires.

There are three forms of vitamin D:

- ✔ *Calciferol* occurs naturally in fish oils and egg yolk; in the United States, manufacturers add it to margarines and milk.

- ✔ *Cholecalciferol* is created when sunlight hits your skin and ultraviolet rays react with steroid chemicals in the body fat just underneath the skin.

- ✔ *Ergocalciferol* is synthesized in plants exposed to sunlight.

Cholecalciferol and ergocalciferol justify vitamin D's nickname: "The sunshine vitamin." The best food sources of vitamin D are fatty fish, such as salmon, or milk. In the United States, all milk is fortified with D.

Vitamin E

Vitamin E keeps your reproductive system humming.

You get your vitamin E from *tocopherols* and *tocotrienols,* two families of chemicals that occur naturally in vegetable oils, nuts, and whole grains. Tocopherols, the more important source, have two sterling characteristics: They're antioxidants and anticoagulants.

The most active tocopherol is alpha-tocopherol, so vitamin E is measured in milligrams of alpha-tocopherol, abbreviated mg-TE.

Vitamin K

Vitamin K is a group of chemicals that your body uses to make specialized proteins found in *blood plasma* (the clear fluid in blood). Among them: *Prothrombin,* the protein chiefly responsible for blood clotting. You also need vitamin K to make bone and kidney tissues.

Vitamin K is found in greens, but your primary source of K is the factory run by friendly intestinal bacteria who churn it out right in your body.

Water-soluble vitamins

The water-soluble vitamins include C and all those busy B's. Because these vitamins dissolve in water, excesses are eliminated in urine. You can't store water-soluble vitamins. You must replace them every day or so.

Vitamin C

Vitamin C, also known as *ascorbic acid,* is essential for the development and maintenance of *connective tissue* (the fat, muscle, and bone framework of the human body). This nutrient is an *antioxidant,* a compound that keeps molecular fragments called free radicals from hooking up with other fragments to form damaging compounds that may attack your tissues (the inside of your blood vessels, for example). Finally, vitamin C protects the immune system, helps you fight off infection, and reduces the severity of allergic reactions.

The best sources of vitamin C are fresh fruits and veggies, like the aforementioned OJ.

Thiamin (vitamin B_1)

Thiamin — known as B_1 because it was the first of the B vitamins that scientists isolated and identified — helps ensure a healthy appetite. It acts as a *co-enzyme* (a substance that works along with an enzyme) essential to at least four different ways that your body extracts energy from carbohydrates. And it's also a mild diuretic.

The best naturally occurring sources of thiamin are pork and pork products; in the United States, all grain products are fortified with B vitamins, including thiamin.

Riboflavin (vitamin B₂)

Riboflavin, the second B vitamin that scientists identified, is essential for the *metabolism* of proteins and carbohydrates (converting these nutrients to energy or new body tissues). Like vitamin A, riboflavin protects the health of mucous membranes, the moist tissues lining eyes, mouth, nose, throat, vagina, and rectum.

The best naturally occurring source of riboflavin is liver; in the United States, all grain products are fortified with B vitamins, including riboflavin.

Niacin

Niacin (a collective name for nicotinic acid and nicotinamide) ensures proper growth, and like other B vitamins, is intimately involved in enzyme reactions. Like thiamin, niacin protects your appetite. Like riboflavin, it takes part in metabolism — in this case, digestion of sugars and fat.

Lamb, chicken, and fish are good natural sources of niacin; in the United States, all grain products are fortified with B vitamins, including niacin.

Pyridoxine (vitamin B₆)

Vitamin B_6 is a component of enzymes that metabolize proteins and fats. Vitamin B_6 is found naturally in bananas, prunes, and plantains, as well as meat and poultry. In the United States, all grain products are fortified with B vitamins, including B_6.

Folate

Folate helps to break dietary proteins apart into their basic components, the amino acids, and then uses these building blocks to create new body cells and tissues. As a result, folate is vital for normal growth, as well as wound healing and the creation of new fetal and maternal tissue during pregnancy. Folate is also a heart-healthy nutrient that helps reduce the risk of *coronary artery disease* (CAD) — heart attack.

The best natural sources of folate are fresh fruits and vegetables, specifically greens. In the United States, all multivitamin supplements have to contain 400 mcg of folate.

Vitamin B₁₂ (cyanocobalamin)

Vitamin B_{12} builds red blood cells, protects *myelin* (the fatty material that covers your nerves), and facilitates the transmission of *electrical impulses* (messages) between nerve cells.

Vitamin B_{12} occurs naturally in dairy foods, meat, fish, and poultry, and, as with vitamin K, those beneficial bacteria in your small intestine make it, too.

Choline

Choline isn't a vitamin, mineral, protein, carbohydrate, or fat, but it's usually lumped in with the B vitamins . . . so heeeeere's choline! In 1998, 138 years after scientists identified choline, the Institute of Medicine (IOM) finally declared it essential for human beings. Your body uses choline to make *acetylcholine,* a chemical that enables brain cells to exchange messages. It protects the heart and lowers the risk of liver cancer, too.

Food sources of choline include eggs, meat, and milk.

Biotin

Biotin, a component of the enzymes that ferry carbon and oxygen atoms between cells, plays a role in metabolizing fats and carbohydrates and is essential for synthesizing fatty acids and amino acids you need for healthy growth.

The best food sources of biotin are liver, egg yolks, yeast, nuts, and grains. If your diet doesn't give you all the biotin you need, those friendly bugs in your gut can take some time off from making K and B_{12} to synthesize extra biotin.

Pantothenic acid

Pantothenic acid, another B vitamin, is vital to enzyme reactions, including the metabolism of carbs and the synthesis of fatty compounds, such as hormones. Pantothenic acid also helps stabilize blood sugar levels, defends against infection, and protects *hemoglobin* (the protein in red blood cells that carries oxygen through the body), as well as nerve, brain, and muscle tissue.

Your best dietary sources of pantothenic acid are meat, fish, poultry, whole grains, and beans. In the United States, all grain products are fortified with B vitamins, including pantothenic acid.

Mining the Minerals

Unlike vitamins (organic compounds made of carbon, hydrogen, and oxygen), *minerals* are inorganic substances composed of only one kind of atom. Another name for minerals is elements.

Minerals occur naturally in nonliving things, such as rocks and metal ores. True, there are minerals in plants and animals, but they're imported. Plants get minerals from soil, and animals get minerals by eating the plants.

Nutritionists classify the minerals essential for human life into one of two categories, depending on how much of the mineral you store in your body and how much you have to consume each day to maintain a steady supply:

- ✔ **Major minerals:** You store more than 5 grams (about one-sixth of an ounce) of each of the major minerals and must take in more than 100 mg a day of each to keep your supply level.

- ✔ **Trace elements:** You store less than 5 grams of each of the trace elements, so you can hold this supply steady with a daily consumption of less than 100 mg of each trace mineral.

Electrolytes: A special kind of mineral

Without enough water in and around its cells, the human body — indeed, any plant or animal — will shrivel up and die. Your body maintains its water level with the help of *electrolytes,* the electrically charged particles called *ions* that are freed when mineral compounds dissolve into their separate parts.

Many minerals, including calcium, phosphorus, and magnesium, form compounds that dissolve into charged particles. But nutritionists generally use the term "electrolyte" to describe three specific major minerals: sodium, potassium, and chlorine. In fact, you're probably most familiar with the source of electrolytes that you can find on virtually every dinner table: sodium chloride. Yes, plain old table salt. In water, sodium chloride breaks apart into two ions, the positively charged (*cation*) sodium ion and the negatively charged (*anion*) chloride ion.

Under normal circumstances, the fluid inside your cells holds more potassium than sodium and chloride. The fluid outside your cells is just the opposite: It holds more sodium and chloride than potassium, but these minerals flow freely back and forth through a process called the *sodium pump.*

If this process stops, sodium ions pile up inside your cells. Sodium attracts water; the more sodium inside the cell, the more water flows in. Eventually, the cell bursts and dies. The sodium pump, regular as a clock, prevents this from happening so that you can sail along, blissfully unconscious of those efficient, electric ions.

Like other nutrients, electrolytes are useful in bodily processes. Sodium helps digest proteins and carbohydrates and smoothes out your pH, so your blood doesn't become too acidic or too basic (alkaline). (For more about pH, check out Chapter 2.) Potassium is also at work in digestion, not to mention the synthesis of proteins and carbs, and as a major constituent of muscle tissue. Chloride is a constituent of *hydrochloric acid,* the gastric juice that helps break down food in your stomach, and white blood cells use it to produce *hypochlorite,* a natural antiseptic. Finally, sodium, potassium, and chloride ions create electrical impulses that enable your cells to zip messages back and forth, making it possible for you to think, see, and move.

Lucky you!

Meeting the majors

The major minerals are calcium, phosphorous, magnesium, sulfur, and the electrolytes sodium, potassium, and chloride.

Although sulfur, a major mineral, is an essential nutrient for human beings, you don't find it listed here — or in most nutrition textbooks. Why? Because sulfur is an integral part of all proteins, so any diet that provides adequate protein also provides adequate sulfur.

Calcium

You know that *calcium* builds strong bones and teeth, reducing your risk of osteoporosis and maybe lowering your dental bills. But do you also know that this mineral helps regulate the amount of water in and around your cells and keeps your muscles from cramping? Or that researchers have recently discovered that a calcium-rich diet may reduce your risk of high blood pressure while lowering your risk of colon cancer by stopping the creation of too many colon cells linked to a high-fat diet? No wonder this is a major mineral!

The best dietary sources of calcium are milk and milk products. There is calcium in some plant foods, such as broccoli, but the calcium is bound tight to other substances, making it hard for your body to grab hold of the calcium.

Phosphorus

Like calcium, *phosphorus* is essential for strong bones and teeth. You also need phosphorous to metabolize carbohydrates, synthesize proteins, and transport fats to your organs and tissues, and protect myelin, the fatty sheath covering each nerve cell. Best of all, phosphorus plays a role in transmitting the *genetic code* (genes and chromosomes that carry information about your special characteristics) from one cell to another when cells divide and reproduce.

The best sources of phosphorous are high protein foods such as meat, fish, poultry, and dairy products.

Magnesium

You need *magnesium* to build body tissues, especially bone; three-quarters of the ounce of magnesium in an adult human body is in the bones. Magnesium is also a constituent of more than 300 different enzymes that trigger the countless chemical reactions throughout your body. And you use magnesium to ship nutrients in and out of body cells, send messages between cells, and — like phosphorous — to transmit your genetic code.

Plant foods, especially bananas and dark green veggies, are good sources of magnesium.

Tracking the traces

Don't be fooled by their name. Trace minerals may sound like small potatoes, but these guys deliver big benefits.

Chromium

Very small amounts of *trivalent chromium,* a digestible form of the shiny metal that decorates your car and household appliances, is essential for building bones and teeth, helping blood clot, regulating your use of glucose, and telegraphing messages back and forth among nerve cells.

Dietary sources of chromium are cereals, meat, fish, poultry, and — three cheers! — beer.

Copper

Copper promotes bone growth, protects nerve cells, enables your body to use iron, and acts as an antioxidant in enzymes that demobilize free radicals and make it possible for your body to use iron. Did I mention it also keeps your hair from turning gray prematurely?

Organ meats (such as liver and heart), seafood, nuts, seeds, and whole grains are natural sources of copper.

Fluoride

Fluoride is the fluorine ion in drinking water. You store fluoride in bones and teeth. Is fluoride an essential nutrient? Nobody knows. But the mineral does harden dental enamel, reducing your risk of cavities, and some researchers suspect (but can't prove) that some forms of fluoride strengthen bones.

Fluoride occurs naturally in some ground water supplies in the western part of the United States, but the common source is artificially fluoridated water.

Iron

Iron is an essential constituent of two pigmented proteins, *hemoglobin* and *myoglobin.* The first carries oxygen around your body; the second stores oxygen in your muscles. Iron is also part of various enzymes that facilitate body chemistry.

The best naturally occurring source of this mineral is *heme* iron, the form of iron found in food from animals (meat, fish, poultry, and dairy products). *Non-heme* iron, the form of iron found in plants, is more difficult to absorb.

Iodine

Iodine is a component of thyroid hormones that regulate chemical processes inside body cells and play an essential role in the synthesis of proteins, the formation and growth of healthy nerves and bones, and the functions of the reproductive system.

Iodine occurs naturally in saltwater fish and plants grown near the ocean, but most Americans get theirs from iodized salt.

Manganese

Manganese, an essential constituent of the enzymes that metabolize carbohydrates and synthesize fats (including cholesterol), is vital for a healthy reproductive system. During pregnancy, it speeds the proper growth of fetal tissue, particularly bones and cartilage.

You find manganese in nuts, beans, whole grains, and tea.

Molybdenum

You need *molybdenum* to build several enzymes that metabolize proteins.

Foods containing molybdenum include nuts, grains, and beans.

Selenium

Selenium regulates thyroid hormones. Like vitamin C it's an antioxidant.

You find selenium in organ meats, seafood, and plants grown in high-selenium soil.

Zinc

Zinc insures healthy growth, protects nerve and brain tissue, and strengthens the immune system. It's a constituent of digestive enzymes and hormones, but most of the zinc in any male body is in the testes, where zinc is used to make a continuing supply of testosterone, the male hormone.

Yes, oysters dish up zinc. So do meat, liver, and eggs. Sounds like a neat lunch.

Brushing up on the bit players

The minerals arsenic, boron, nickel, silicon, and vanadium are special cases. Nutritionists think these elements are useful, but nobody know exactly what they do. Sooner or later, someone will find out what role these minerals play in nutrition. For now, no RDA/AI exist for these nutrients, but some are clearly hazardous to your health in large amounts. Hey, arsenic comes quickly to mind, right?

Sizing up the megadose mystery

What's a megadose? By general consensus, the word means an amount of a nutrient several times the RDA/AI. But in fact, the term is so vague that I can't find it in either my medical dictionary or the dictionary on my computer.

Nonetheless, it's perfectly clear that very big doses of vitamins and minerals can wreak havoc in your body. The easiest way to avoid these problems is to stick to the RDAs. What problems, you may ask. Well, for example:

✔ Excess vitamin A may cause liver damage, abnormal vision, and symptoms similar to those of a brain tumor. Worse yet, amounts usually considered normal may be problematic. A 30-year study at University Hospital in Uppsala (Sweden) shows that 5,000 IU vitamin A, the amount found in virtually all basic multivitamin tablets, may inhibit the production of new bone cells, increase the loss of existing bone, and make it hard for vitamin D to push calcium into bone. The result: An up to 700 percent increase in the risk of hip fractures among older people. To counter this effect, the Swedish scientists recommend changing the RDA from the current 3,000 IU for everyone to 3,000 IU for men and 2,400 IU for women.

✔ Overdosing on iron supplements can be deadly, especially for young children. The lethal dose for a young child may be as low as 3 grams (3,000 mg) elemental iron, the amount in 60 tablets with 50 mg elemental iron each. For adults, the lethal dose is estimated to be 200 to 250 mg elemental iron per kilogram (2.2 pounds) of body weight. That's about 13,600 mg for a 150-pound person, the amount you'd get in 292 tablets with 50 mg elemental iron each, an amount you're really unlikely to swallow by mistake.

✔ Doses of molybdenum 2 to 7 times the AI increase your loss of copper in urine.

✔ Chinese nutrition researchers have linked doses as high as 5 mg selenium a day (70 to 99 times the RDA) to thickened but fragile nails, hair loss, and garlicky perspiration. In the United States, a small group of people who had accidentally gotten a supplement mistakenly containing 27.3 mg selenium (400 to 500 times the RDA) ended up with *selenium intoxication* — fatigue, abdominal pain, nausea, diarrhea, and nerve damage.

✔ Moderately high doses of zinc (up to 25 mg a day) can make it hard for your body to absorb copper. Doses 20 times the 15 mg RDA interfere with your immune function and make you more susceptible to infection, the very thing that normal doses of zinc protect against. Gram doses (2,000 mg/2 grams) of zinc trigger zinc poisoning: vomiting, gastric upset, and irritation of the stomach lining.

Which brings me back to the beginning: What's a megadose? Sorry, the amounts listed above are clearly unhealthy, but nobody's labeled them with the M word.

Supplementing the Info

The argument over the value of *dietary supplements* (vitamins, minerals, and other nutrients) has swung back and forth so often that you could get whiplash trying to follow it. Today, most experts agree that most people can get the nutrition they need from food, but others may need extra help from supplements.

Who are these other folks that may need to take supplements? The obvious candidates are women of childbearing age. Simply adding a daily supplement containing 400 mcg of folate has now been proven to dramatically reduce the risk of birth defects of the spinal cord. Women who are pregnant need additional amounts of nutrients to protect a growing fetus. Women who are nursing need extra nutrients to produce sufficient amounts of milk.

And don't forget:

- ✔ People taking medicines that increase or decrease the effectiveness of vitamins and minerals. For example, taking aspirin on a regular basis may reduce absorption of vitamin C; using diuretics may reduce calcium absorption.

- ✔ People who smoke (What? There are still people who smoke?) need extra vitamin C. The current RDA is 100 mg for smokers, 10 mg higher than the RDA for men who don't smoke and 25 mg higher than the RDA for women who don't smoke.

- ✔ People who follow a *vegan diet*. This diet is the purest form of vegetarianism, excluding all foods from animals, including dairy foods. Without milk products, vegans may not get the vitamin D that they need. Because the iron in plants is more difficult to absorb than the iron in animal foods, they may also need iron supplements.

- ✔ Women of childbearing age may need extra iron to replace the iron lost in menstrual bleeding; men may need zinc to replace the mineral they lose in ejaculate.

As for you and your reflux, do you need supplements? The unequivocal answer is: It depends. If your reflux rules out whole categories of foods, such as fresh fruits, then yes, you may need supplements. If only a few foods are off your personal menu — for example, you can't tolerate oranges, but tomatoes and grapefruit are fine — no, you may not need supplements. Only your doctor knows for sure. So ask her.

Crunching the numbers

Don't want to sit through a learn-your-vitamins-and-minerals session with your doctor? Then go right ahead and check out Table 5-2 and Table 5-3, which lay out the latest vitamin and mineral recommendations for healthy teens and adults. Some of these numbers are RDAs; others are AIs (adequate intakes). Either way, they are what a healthy body needs to stay in tiptop form.

Table 5-2	Vitamins and Minerals: The RDAs

g = gram   R = retinol
mg = milligram   a-TE = alpha-tocopherol equivalent
mcg = microgram   NE = niacin equivalent

Age (Years)	Vitamin A (mcgRE)	Vitamin D (mcg/IU)	Vitamin E (mg/a-TE)	Vitamin K (mcg)	Vitamin C (mg)
Infants/Children					
0.0–0.5	400	5/200	4*	2*	40*
0.5–1.0	500	5/200	5*	2.5*	50*
1–3	300	5/200	6	30*	15
4–8	400	5/200	7	55*	25
Males					
9–13	600	5/200	11	60*	45
14–18	900	5/200	15	75*	75
19–30	900	5/200	15	120*	90
31–50	900	5/200	15	120*	90
51–70	900	10/400	15	120*	90
Older than 70	900	15/600	15	120*	90
Females					
9–13	600	5/200	11	60*	45
14–18	700	5/200	15	75*	65
19–30	700	5/200	15	90*	76
31–50	700	5/200	15	90*	75
51–70	700	10/400	15	90*	75
Older than 70	700	15/500	15	90*	75
Pregnant	750–770	5/200	15	75–90*	70
Nursing	1,200–1,300	5/200	19	76–90*	95

*AI/adequate intake
* *The new AI for people age 71 and older is 15mcg/600 IU.

(continued)

Table 5-2 *(continued)*

g	=	gram	R	=	retinol
mg	=	milligram	a-TE	=	alpha-tocopherol equivalent
mcg	=	microgram	NE	=	niacin equivalent

Age (Years)	Thiamin (Vitamin B₁) (mg)	Riboflavin (Vitamin B₂) (mg)	Niacin (mcg/NE)	Vitamin B₆ (mg)	Folate (mcg)	Vitamin B₁₂ (mcg)
Infants/Children						
0.0–0.5	0.2*	0.3*	2*	0.1*	65*	0.4*
0.5–1.0	0.3*	0.45*	46*	0.3*	80*	0.5*
1–3	0.5	0.5	6	0.5	150	0.9
4–8	0.6	0.6	8	0.6	200	1.2
Males						
9–13	0.9	0.9	12	1.0	300	1.8
14–18	1.2	1.3	16	1.2	400	2.4
19–30	1.2	1.3	16	1.3	400	2.4
31–50	1.2	1.3	16	1.3	400	2.4
51–70	1.2	1.3	16	1.7	400	2.4
Older than 70	1.2	1.3	16	1.7	400	2.4
Females						
9–13	0.9	0.9	12	1.0	300	1.8
14–18	1.0	1.0	14	1.2	400	2.4
19–30	1.1	1.1	14	1.3	400	2.4
31–50	1.1	1.1	14	1.3	400	2.4
51–70	1.1	1.1	14	1.5	400	2.4
Older than 70	1.1	1.1	14	1.5	400	2.4
Pregnant	1.4	1.1	18	1.9	600	2.6
Nursing	1.4	1.1	17	2.0	500	2.8

Age (years)	Calcium (mg)	Phosphorus (mg)	Magnesium (mg)	Iron (mg)	Zinc (mg)
Infants/Children					
0.0–0.5	210*	100*	30*	0.27*	2*
0.5–1.0	270*	275*	75*	11	3
1–3	500*	460	80	7	3
4–8	800*	500	130	10	5

Age (Years)	Calcium (mg)	Phosphorus (mg)	Magnesium (mg)	Iron (mg)	Zinc (mg)
Males					
9–13	1,300*	1,250	240	8	8
14–18	1,300*	1,250	410	11	11
19–30	1,000*	700	400	8	11
31–50	1,000*	700	420	8	11
51–70	1,200*	700	420	8	11
Older than 70	1,200*	700	420	8	11
Females					
9–13	1,300*	1,250	240	8	82
14–18	1,300*	1,250	360	15	92
19–30	1,000*	700	310	18	8
31–50	1,000*	700	320	18	8
51–70	1,200*	700	700	320	8
Older than 70	1,200*	700	320	8	8
Pregnant	1,000–1,300*	700–1,250	350–400	27	11–12
Nursing	1,000–1,300*	700–1,250	310–350	9–10	12–13

* Adequate Intake (AI)

Age (Years)	Iodine (mcg)	Selenium (mcg)	Molybdenum (mcg)
Infants/Children			
0.0–0.5	110*	15*	2*
0.5–1.0	130*	20*	3*
1–3	90	20	17
4–8	90	30	22
Males			
9–13	120	40	34
14–18	150	55	43
19–30	150	55	45
31–50	150	55	45
51–70	150	55	45
Older than 70	150	55	45

*Adequate intake (AI)

(continued)

Table 5-2 *(continued)*

g	=	gram	R	=	retinol
mg	=	milligram	a-TE	=	alpha-tocopherol equivalent
mcg	=	microgram	NE	=	niacin equivalent

Age (Years)	Iodine (mcg)	Selenium (mcg)	Molybdenum (mcg)
Females			
9–13	120	40	34
14–18	150	55	43
19–30	150	55	45
31–50	150	55	45
51–70	150	55	45
Older than 70	150	55	45
Pregnant	220	60	50
Nursing	290	70	50

*Adequate intake (AI)

Table 5-3 — Adequate Intake (AI)

Age (Years)	Biotin (mcg)	Pantothenic Acid (mg)	Copper (mcg)	Manganese (mg)	Fluoride (mg)
Infants/Children					
0.0–0.5	5	1.7	200	0.003	0.01
0.5–1.0	6	1.8	220	0.6	0.5
1–3	8	2	340	1.2	0.7
4–8	12	3–4	440	1.5	1
Males					
9–13	20	4	700	1.9	2
14–18	25	5	890	2.2	3
19–30	30	5	900	2.3	4
31–50	30	5	900	2.3	4
51–70	30	5	900	2.3	4
Older than 70	30	5	900	2.3	4
Females					
9–13	20	4	700	1.6	2
14–18	25	5	890	1.6	3

Age (Years)	Biotin (mcg)	Pantothenic Acid (mg)	Copper (mcg)	Manganese (mg)	Fluoride (mg)
19–30	30	5	900	1.8	3
31–50	30	5	900	1.8	3
51–70	30	5	900	1.8	3
Older than 70	30	5	900	1.8	3
Pregnant	30	6	1,000	2.0	1.5–4.0
Nursing	35	7	1,300	2.6	1.5–4.0

Age (Years)	Chromium (mcg)	Choline (mg)
Infants/Children		
0.0–0.5	0.2	125
0.5–1.0	5.5	150
1–3	11	200
4–8	15	250
Males		
9–13	25	375
14–18	35	550
19–30	36	550
31–50	36	550
51–70	30	550
Older than 70	30	550
Females		
9–13	21	375
14–18	24	400
19–30	25	425
31–50	25	425

Age (Years)	Chromium (mcg)	Choline (mg)
51–70	20	425
Older than 70	20	425
Pregnant	29–30	450
Nursing	44–45	550

Source: Adapted with permission from Recommended Dietary Allowances (Washington D.C.: National Academy Press, 1989, and DRI panel reports)

Setting limits

Some folks just don't know when to quit so the National Academy of Medicine's Food and Nutrition Board has set a Tolerable Upper Limit (UL) to give you a good idea of what's safe when taking vitamins and minerals. Table 5-4 shows the current ULs for vitamins and minerals. Ain't that handy? (See the sidebar "Sizing up the megadose mystery" in this chapter for more info on going too far with vitamins and minerals.) Wait! Right now there are no ULs set for K, B_1, B_2, B_{12}, biotin, and pantothenic acid. Sorry about that!

Table 5-4	Setting Upper Limits for Vitamins and Minerals*
Nutrient	*UL (Tolerable Upper Limit)***
Vitamins	
Vitamin A	3,000 mcg
Vitamin D	50 mcg
Vitamin E	1,000 mg
Vitamin B_6	100 mg
Choline	3,500 mg
Folate	1,000 mcg
Niacin	35 mg
Vitamin C	2,000 mg
Minerals	
Calcium	2,500 mg
Phosphorus	4,000 mg
Magnesium	350 mg
Chromium	35 for men age 19-50
	30 for men older than 50
	25 for women age 19–50
	20 for women older than 50
Copper	10,000 mcg
Fluoride	10 mg
Iodine	1,100 mcg
Iron	45 mg

Nutrient	UL (Tolerable Upper Limit)**
Manganese	11 mg
Molybdenum	45 mcg
Selenium	400 mcg
Zinc	40 mg
Boron	20 mg
Nickel	1.0 mg
Vanadium	1.8 mg

*The Food and Nutrition Board hasn't established ULs for vitamin K, thiamin, riboflavin, B_{12}, biotin, pantothenic acid, and chromium.

**Unless otherwise noted, these ULs are for healthy men and women age 19–70.

Source: Academy of Medicine Food and Nutrition Board

Chapter 6

Fine-Tuning Your Diet

*T*his chapter gets right to the meat of the matter: How to eat well and keep your tummy comfy at the same time. First, I talk about the pleasure of dining well. Next, I provide a guide to the foods most likely to trigger acid reflux either by weakening your lower esophageal sphincter (LES) or by irritating your esophagus. Then, I offer a plan on how to find out which foods are your own personal problematics. And for the windup, I share a sensible cook's tour of cooking methods.

Know in advance that this chapter is a list-maker's delight, with whole bunches of charts and tables. Why? Because assembling a list of heartburn triggers takes up a lot less space than putting the information into long paragraphs. Do your eyes glaze over at the sight of columns of words? Relax. Take them *slowly,* one at a time. Finally, don't forget to check out Chapter 5 to see how the foods and beverages in this chapter can fit into a nutritious diet. And now on to the main event: Breakfast. Lunch. Dinner.

Enjoying Food

The *Dietary Guidelines for Americans* is a down-to-earth, totally sensible collection of rules on how to eat well from your friends at the U.S. Departments of Agriculture and Health and Human Services, hereinafter referred to as the party of the first part . . . no, no, just kidding. I use their initials: USDA and HHS.

The *Dietary Guidelines for Americans* lays out food and lifestyle choices that not only promote good health and provide the energy you need for an active life but may also go a long way toward reducing your risk of chronic illnesses such as diabetes and heart disease. You can access the guidelines online at www.health.gov/dietaryguidelines.

If you've never actually seen the guidelines, know that my book *Nutrition For Dummies* (Wiley) covers them up, down, and sideways, with detailed comments on every single point made by the USDA and HHS. For the moment, I zero in on a sentence in the very first paragraph on the very first page of the guidelines:

"Eating is one of life's greatest pleasures."

Instead of relishing one of life's pleasures, people with heartburn often look at a well-appointed dinner plate with a mixture of fear and trembling. "Will that juice light my reflux fire?" they wonder. "How about the salad? the burger? the cheese? the pie?" Sad to say, their worry is often well founded. Some foods *do* cause reflux and heartburn. But the question is

- ✔ How does heartburn happen?
- ✔ Which foods are to blame?
- ✔ How can you identify the ones most likely to bite back when you bite them?

Come to think of it, that's three questions. Today's your lucky day. I answer each question in the following sections.

Explaining How Food and Drink Can Cause Heartburn

The food you eat and the beverages you drink may raise your risk of heartburn by

- ✔ Increasing the number of times you experience reflux
- ✔ Making stomach contents more acidic so that any reflux is more painful
- ✔ Irritating the lining of your esophagus on the way down, even without triggering reflux

Read the next section to discover the foods and drinks to blame for each of these events.

Weakening the LES

When you're talking heartburn, the center of action is always LES, the trap-door between the esophagus and stomach that closes tight after you've swallowed food to keep acidic stomach contents from washing back, or *refluxing,* into your esophagus. If the LES opens accidentally, allowing acidic stomach contents to wash back into your esophagus, you get heartburn. If reflux were a crime, the likely perps may be the foods and beverages in the next sections.

High-fat foods

Your body digests fat more slowly than it digests proteins and carbohydrates, which is why you feel full longer after eating a high-fat filet mignon or a chopped chuck burger than after feasting on a skin-free chicken breast or a lettuce-and-tomato salad with low-fat dressing.

Don't dive into your martini

Add up all the pros and cons about alcohol beverages, and you can plainly see that moderate drinking confers the most benefits with the fewest risks. For some people with severe heartburn, moderate may be as little as one drink a year on New Year's Eve. For others, the standards from the *Dietary Guidelines for Americans* may apply. The guidelines define moderate drinking as one drink a day for a woman, two drinks a day for a man. What's a drink? 1.5 ounces spirits, 5 ounces wine, 12 ounces beer — the amount of alcohol one healthy adult human body can metabolize in one to two hours.

But "nowadays" — to quote those perky *Chicago* gunslingers Roxie Hart and Velma Kelley — these numbers can seem puny when you eyeball the drinks at your local Hot Stuff Bar. Depending on the drink, the bartender may be pouring anywhere from 3 ounces of your favorite spirit (plus 3 ounces mixer) to as much as 6 ounces tequila, vodka, gin . . . the list goes on . . . into the swimming-pool–size glass shown in the following figure. If one of these drinks ends up in front of you, regardless of your heartburn status, look carefully before you leap. Then don't leap. Period.

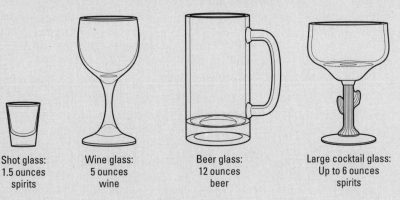

Shot glass:
1.5 ounces
spirits

Wine glass:
5 ounces
wine

Beer glass:
12 ounces
beer

Large cocktail glass:
Up to 6 ounces
spirits

A full stomach exerts pressure against the LES. The longer the stomach is full, the longer the pressure lasts. Anyone see trouble looming?

Alcohol beverages

Beer, wine, and spirits increase your risk of reflux-related heartburn in two distinct ways.

- First, alcohol is the muscle-relaxant *par excellence,* which is French for, "nothing better than this one, kid." The LES is a muscle. Alcohol relaxes muscles. See the reflux connection?

- Second, alcohol is an acidic liquid. Alcohol beverages can trigger the production of excess acid in your stomach, and they're perfectly capable of annoying your esophagus on the way down, even before they bounce back as reflux.

In 1997, a report featured in the medical journal *Digestive Disease Sciences* said that people who drink about 12 ounces of red wine at lunch or dinner have higher than normal levels of acid in their esophagi (never say esophaguses!) and are exposed to high acidity up to four times longer than diners who quaffed tap water. Similar results are linked to the other forms of alcohol beverages. Does that mean a person with heartburn may never again indulge in a cup of good cheer — or a simple glass of beer, wine, or spirits? The straightforward, forthright, no-waffle is, *it depends.*

If the slightest sniff of the cork sets off your reflux, pass the bottle. But if one drink every once in a while feels fine, the National Heartburn Alliance (NHBA) says, enjoy. In other words — heartburn or no heartburn — when the subject is alcohol, the watchwords are *good sense* and *moderation.* Read more about drinking in the sidebar "Don't dive into your martini" in this chapter.

Carbonated beverages

Carbonated beverages get their bounce from carbon dioxide, a gas that keeps bubbling even after it enters your stomach. Imagine all those teeny little carbon dioxide bubbles bumping up against your LES, pushing and shoving and — what more can I say?

Well, the word "burp" comes quickly to mind, as in the sound of air forcing itself up through the LES into your esophagus — and almost certainly carrying acid reflux along with it. And if that's not bad enough, imagine what happens when you mix some alcohol with those bubbles.

Making more acid

Virtually any combination of food cobbled together in a large meal sends a direct order to your stomach: "Lots of stuff here," it says. "Send out more acid to digest it."

The larger your meal and the more high-fat foods it contains, the higher the amount of acid your stomach must churn out to digest it all. Are you really surprised to hear that large meals — especially those high in fat — are more likely than small meals to cause reflux?

Irritating your esophagus

Like some people, some foods and beverages are just plain annoying, so acidic on their own that they irritate your esophagus even in the absence of acid reflux. Three common acid troublemakers are

- Alcohol beverages (with or without mixers and juices)
- Citrus fruits and juices (including tomatoes)
- Coffee, that perennial heartburn trigger — as in plain java, espresso, cappuccino, low-fat mocha, and so on! How sad!

Naming the Guilty Parties

Okay, so now you know that some foods can loosen your LES, make your stomach churn out more acid, or scratch up your esophagus. But exactly which foods?

Well, I'm glad you asked because I've been sitting here, waiting impatiently, to introduce you to a neat set of tables, which list foods that are good, foods that occupy the middle ground, and foods that are Big Trouble. And I also have a few good ways for you to identify and track your own personal Big Trouble foods.

Deciphering the rules of the road

When you get behind the wheel of your wheels, your brain immediately assigns a specific meaning to three otherwise pretty but pretty meaningless colors:

- Go on **green.**
- Slow down on **yellow.**
- Stop on **red.**

The NHBA used the same color code when choosing a diet to reduce the risk of heartburn. The NHBA *Stop and Select Guide* is a color-coded chart that rates many foods and beverages on their tendency to give you heartburn or make reflux worse. Just like a traffic light, the chart means the following:

✔ **Green means go:** This food is unlikely to cause heartburn or make it worse.

✔ **Yellow means slow down:** If you're going to eat this food, make sure you don't overdo.

✔ **Red means stop:** This food often causes heartburn. Do you really want it on your plate?

TIP

To see the full-color Stop and Select chart online, visit www. heartburnalliance.org, click on the link for free brochures, and follow the prompts. If you're not into the Internet, you can order a copy by dialing 877-642-2453. Snail mailers can get one by writing The National Heartburn Alliance, 303 East Wacker Drive, Suite 418, Chicago, Illinois 60601.

You can also run an inquisitive finger down Tables 6-1, 6-2, 6-3, and 6-4 right now to see what foods are Green, Yellow, and Red. (The foods are grouped according to standard USDA food pyramid groupings.)

Table 6-1	Fruits and Veggies
Fruits	*Vegetables*
R: Orange juice	**R:** Mashed potatoes
R: Lemon	**R:** French fries
R: Lemonade	**R:** Onion, raw
R: Grapefruit juice	**R:** Potato salad
R: Cranberry juice	**Y:** Garlic
R: Tomato	**Y:** Onion, cooked
Y: Low-acid orange juice	**Y:** Leeks
Y: Apple cider	**Y:** Sauerkraut
Y: Peach	**Y:** Scallions
Y: Blueberries	**G:** Carrots
Y: Raspberries	**G:** Cabbage
Y: Strawberries	**G:** Peas
Y: Grapes	**G:** Broccoli
Y: Cranberries, dried	**G:** Green beans
G: Apple	**G:** Baked potato
G: Apple juice	
G: Banana	

Source: The Stop and Select Guide is provided by the National Heartburn Alliance.

Table 6-2	Bread and Butter
Grains	*Dairy*
R: Macaroni and cheese	**R:** Sour cream
R: Spaghetti with marinara sauce	**R:** Milkshake
Y: Garlic bread	**R:** Ice cream
Y: Muffin	**R:** Cottage cheese, regular
Y: Granola cereal	**Y:** Yogurt
G: Multigrain bread	**Y:** Milk, 2 percent
G: White bread	**Y:** Milk, skim
G: Corn bread	**Y:** Frozen yogurt
G: Brown rice	**Y:** Cottage cheese, low-fat
G: White rice	**Y:** Cheddar cheese
G: Couscous	**Y:** Mozzarella cheese
G: Graham crackers	**G:** Cream cheese, fat-free
G: Saltine crackers	**G:** Feta cheese
G: Pretzels	**G:** Goat cheese
G: Rice cakes	**G:** Sour cream, fat-free
G: Oatmeal cereal	**G:** Soy cheese, low-fat
G: Frosted cereal	
G: Bran-based cereal	

Source: The Stop and Select Guide is provided by the National Heartburn Alliance.

Table 6-3	Meats, Beans, and Other Proteins
Meats	*Beans and Other Proteins*
R: Ground beef, chuck	**Y:** Scrambled eggs, in butter
R: Marble sirloin	**Y:** Eggs, fried
R: Chicken, nugget style	**Y:** Nuts or peanut butter
R: Chicken, buffalo wings	**Y:** Baked beans

(continued)

Table 6-3 *(continued)*

Meats	Beans and Other Proteins
Y: Ground beef, lean	**G:** Egg whites/egg substitute
Y: Chicken salad	
Y: Tuna salad	
Y: Hot dog, beef or pork	
Y: Ham	
G: Ground beef, extra lean	
G: Steak, London broil	
G: Chicken breast, without skin	
G: Fish, fresh, prepared without added fat	

Source: The Stop and Select Guide is provided by the National Heartburn Alliance.

Table 6-4   Fun Food

Fats, Oils, and Sweets	Beverages
R: Chocolate	**R:** Liquor (spirits)
R: Corn chips	**R:** Wine
R: Potato chips, regular	**R:** Coffee
R: Butter cookie, high fat	**R:** Tea
R: Brownie	**Y:** Non-alcoholic, wine
R: Doughnut	**Y:** Beer
R: Salad dressing, creamy	**Y:** Non-alcoholic beer
Y: Cookie, low-fat	**Y:** Cola
Y: Ketchup	**Y:** Root beer
G: Potato chips, baked	**G:** Mineral water
G: Cookie, fat-free	
G: Jelly beans	
G: Red licorice	
G: Salad dressing, low-fat	

Source: The Stop and Select Guide is provided by the National Heartburn Alliance.

Shaking up the spice rack

Herbs and spices and condiments, such as ketchup and mayonnaise, add zest to food. But do they add heat to the fire in your esophagus? It depends on the herb, spice, or condiment.

For hundreds of years, the word *herb* was reserved for leafy seasonings like parsley and thyme, while the word spice was used for hard or woody seasonings such as peppercorns, nutmeg, or cinnamon bark. Today, in the interest of simplicity, most people refer to virtually every plant product that seasons food as an herb.

Whether an herb makes your heartburn bloom depends on which herb you're using. As a general rule — riddled with exceptions — the "cool greens" are less likely than "hot" seasonings to be troublesome. In addition, some seasonings, such as onions and garlic, are less troublesome dried than fresh. (For more on herbs used as home remedies, check out Chapter 7.) The following herbs are *less* likely to cause heartburn:

- Basil
- Cinnamon
- Coriander
- Dill
- Garlic powder
- Ginger (ground)
- Mace (ground)
- Onion powder, dried onion
- Parsley
- Tarragon
- Thyme

On the other hand, according to the NHBA, the following herbs are *more* likely to cause heartburn:

- Black pepper
- Chili powder
- Cloves
- Curry powder
- Garlic, fresh

✔ Mint

✔ Mustard seed

✔ Nutmeg

✔ Pepper — black, red (hot), white

These lists are a tentative guide, because just as some people can slide off to dreamland after umpteen cups of high-octane regular coffee, others can down a ton of red-hot jalapeños without so much as an "ouch." (Check out the next section, "Identifying your personal troublemakers," which shows you how to identify your own personal problematic foods and beverages.)

As for basic condiments,

✔ **Ketchup's** just another way to say *tomato sauce.* If you have no problems with the former, the latter is probably peachy keen. And vice versa, too.

✔ **Mayonnaise** may be less troublesome in low-fat or no-fat versions. Ditto for salad dressings.

✔ **Mustard** is iffy — all that vinegar (see the next entry) and irritating mashed mustard seed.

✔ **Vinegar** is a high-acid liquid that sounds like a definite Don't Touch. But for some unknown reason, some people seem to find *cider vinegar* and *rice vinegar* less irritating than *white vinegars* (including the flavored versions). Only your own esophagus knows for sure.

Identifying your personal troublemakers

No matter how many individual scientists or health groups classify foods as green, red, yellow, hot, or cool as to their ability to stir up heartburn among the general population, individual bodies often beg to differ. Gastro gurus really do know which foods raise red flags most often, but they can never know for sure which foods will misbehave in which people's bodies.

So guess what? You're about to become your own personal research study. You can use a *Heartburn Food Diary* to keep tabs on the foods that set your reflux alarm bells ringing. The process is simple: Every time you eat or drink something, you record it in the diary. It's a simple way to track the effect of specific foods and beverages on your risk of heartburn. Check out the sample page from a completed Heartburn Food Diary in Table 6-5. For the best results, keep a diary for a week or two or even a month to provide a broad sampling and repeated trials of various foods.

Get out a notebook and create the five columns you see in Table 6-5. Or photocopy the diary page in Figure 6-1. Make one copy for each day you keep the diary.

Heartburn Food Diary

Day	Time	Food/Beverage	Ouch! Index (0-3)	Ouch! Index One Hour Later (0-3)

Figure 6-1:
Dear
diary . . . .

Here's how to use the Heartburn Food Diary:

1. **For your first entry, record the day and time for your first meal.**

   Or, if you're the type that skips breakfast, proper, make a day/time entry for the first time you eat or drink anything.

2. **In the Food/Beverage column, list all the foods and beverages you consume at that setting, being as accurate as possible.**

   For example, if you have buttered toast, don't just write *toast;* write *buttered toast.* If you have one small cup of coffee, write *coffee, small cup.* If you have the super-sized version, write *coffee, 20 ounces.* Or you can just write *big coffee.*

   The point is that being as descriptive as possible makes analyzing your diary — with the goal of making food choices that reduce your risk of heartburn — more productive. A single small cup of java may not upset your insides, but a large one may give you heartburn. If you're in this position and you love coffee, knowing that limiting, not necessarily reducing, your coffee consumption will be welcome news.

3. **Fill in the Ouch! Index column.**

   The Ouch! Index is a scale of how much pain you feel after eating or drinking a specific serving of a specific food or beverage. Use the following rating system:

   0 = This food didn't give me heartburn.

   1 = This food gave me a slight twinge.

   2 = This food gave me moderate heartburn.

   3 = This food gave me such bad heartburn that I'd consider eliminating it from my diet.

4. **An hour later, record a second Ouch! Index reading.**

5. **Repeat Steps 1 through 4 each time you eat or drink anything for the entire day.**

6. **Continue making diary entries for one or two weeks, using a separate page for each day.**

Table 6-5		Sample Heartburn Food Diary Page		
Day	*Time*	*Food/Beverage*	*Ouch! Index (0–3)*	*Ouch! Index One Hour Later*
Monday	8 a.m.	Orange juice, slice of toast	3	2
	11 a.m.	Half bagel, with light cream cheese	0	0
	1 p.m.	Mixed green salad, with low-fat ranch dressing	1	1
	3 p.m.	Large chocolate bar	1	2

After you've completed the diary for a week or two, get out that calculator and put on your math hat to evaluate your food choices according to your diary results. Find another piece of notebook paper, and create the four columns you see in Table 6-6. Your mission is to determine an average Ouch! Index number for each food and beverage from your diary.

1. **Record the first food or beverage you find on Day 1 of your diary.**

   From the example in Table 6-5, that's orange juice.

2. **Record each Ouch! Index number that you find throughout your diary for that particular food.**

   As you can see on Table 6-6, I've recorded seven Ouch! Index numbers for orange juice, meaning I had seven servings over the one-week period.

3. **Add up each individual Ouch! Index number to get a total Ouch! Index number.**

   In Table 6-6, the math is 3 + 3 + 2 + 2 + 3 + 3 + 3 = 19.

4. **Divide the total Ouch! Index number from Step 3 by the number of individual servings you've recorded in Step 2 to arrive at your average Ouch! Index number for that particular food or beverage.**

   You can do either the Instant Ouch! Index or the One Hour Ouch! Index. *Remember:* This is a guide, not an inviolable prediction.

   Round up or down in the usual manner (down for less than 0.5; up for greater than 0.5).

   From Table 6-6, the math is 19 ÷ 7 = 2.7 = 3.

5. **Repeat Steps 1 through 4 until you account for all foods and beverages in your diary.**

6. **Apply the following scale to your average Ouch! Index number:**

   > **0** = This food never gives me heartburn.

   > **1** = This food sometimes gives me heartburn.

   > **2** = This food often gives me heartburn.

   > **3** = This food always gives me heartburn.

7. **Look at the results and draw conclusions.**

   For example: No more "3" foods, occasional servings of "2" foods, frequent servings of "1" foods, as much as you can eat of foods that rank 0 so long as you watch the portion size. But remember that large servings of even the most innocent foods may fan heartburn flames.

8. **Clear your conclusions with your doctor.**

9. **Tailor your food choices to your tummy and feel better.**

Table 6-6	Evaluating My Food Choices	
Food	*Ouch! Index Entries*	*Ouch! Index Average*
Orange juice	3,3,2,2,3,3,3	19 divided by 7 = 2.7 = 3
Bagel	0,0,0,1,0,1,0	2 divided by 7 = 0.3 = 0

Another way to say *warning* is *caveat emptor,* which is Latin for "buyer beware." Say you read all the directions in this section and you fill out the *Heartburn Food Diary* exactly as you're supposed to, even making sure your handwriting is clear enough so that you can actually read it several days from now. If you eat more than one food at the same time, and you have heartburn an hour later, how in the world can you tell which food — the orange juice or the bagel — did you in? Good question. Unfortunately, you may not be able to decipher the results.

Sure, you could eat one food at 8 a.m. another at 9 a.m., and so on through the day and then evaluate the results. But who's kidding whom? The better way is to watch for patterns. If you have heartburn after orange juice and a bagel, no heartburn after a bagel and apple juice, and heartburn again after orange juice and a salad, maybe that's a hint that the problem is the orange juice. The longer you keep your diary, the more accurate the results will be, even though like so much in life, the diary is a guide, not a guarantee.

Making Meals Safer

This section is all good news because no matter how troublesome a food, a drink, or a meal may seem, you may be able to reduce its impact on your risk of heartburn and reflux by adjusting your meal schedule, your eating speed, or the way the food's prepared.

Setting a soothing schedule

What you eat is only one part of your reducing-reflux game plan. When you eat is also an important factor. For example, does your brain translate "three square" into "four courses"? Remember that large meals — especially large meals with lots of fat — increase your risk of reflux. Take a moment to go back to the section "High-fat foods" for a refresher course. Your tummy will say, "Thank you."

Breaking three big meals into several smaller ones is a good idea — as long as one of those extra meals isn't late at night. For more about why eating close to bedtime isn't a good idea, plus several tips on how to sleep heartburn-free, check out Chapter 14.

Slowing down the action

Do people who eat fast gain more weight than people who eat slowly? Nope. But do people who eat fast increase their risk of acid reflux? Yup. To put that concept in terms more scientific than "Yup" and "Nope," I consider what Stephen M. Wildi of the Medical University of South Carolina-Charleston said when addressing the Digestive Disease Week conference in Orlando, Florida in May 2003. The faster you eat, the higher your risk of reflux. I'm paraphrasing, of course, but his point is clear.

Wildi based his conclusion on a study in which researchers asked ten healthy volunteers to eat a normal, 690-calorie meal at two speeds: in five minutes one day, 30 minutes the next. Then the docs carefully observed the diners for two hours after the meal to watch for signs of reflux. (A groan? A grimace? A dash to the antacid bottle?)

The careful observation showed that eating fast produced up to 50 percent more episodes of reflux than eating slowly. The nonscientific conclusion? Mom was right. Don't bolt your food.

Modifying foods and recipes

Sometimes a food's form or the way it's served can make a difference in the likelihood of its triggering your reflux. For example, raw onions are generally a no-no, but dried onion flakes are generally okay. Check out the following simple rules for culinary care:

- ✔ **Grains:** Breads, rice, and pasta are usually user-friendly, but sauces and spreads can be problematic. In general, light broth-based pasta sauces are less irritating than high-fat creamy ones. For bread, opt for low-fat or fat-free spreads.

- ✔ **Seasonings:** Dried or dehydrated is often safer than fresh. For example, dried garlic chips, onion flakes, and green pepper flakes are less irritating than fresh garlic, onions, and green peppers. Alas, absolutely nothing takes the fire away from hot red, black, or white peppers.

- ✔ **Meat, fish, poultry, and egg dishes:** Lower-fat sauce or prep method equals lower heartburn risk.

- ✔ **Oils:** The general rule: A little goes a long way.

Choosing the Safest Cooking Technique

I've always guessed that the first cooked dinner was an accident involving some poor wandering animal and a bolt of lightening that — zap! — charred the beast into medium sirloin. Then, a caveman attracted by the aroma tore off a sizzled hunk, and forthwith offered up the first restaurant rating: "Yum." After that, it was but a hop, a skip, and a jump, anthropologically speaking, to open fires, gas ranges, and electric broilers, enabling human beings to control cooking rather than relying on a passing thunderbolt. Throughout the centuries, human beings have generally relied on three simple methods to heat their food:

- ✔ **An open flame:** You hold the food directly over (or under) the flame or — to avoid sizzling your fingers — you put in a pot on top of the flame or a broiler underneath. ***Note:*** The electric heating coil is simply a modern version of an open flame.

- ✔ **A closed hot box:** You put the food in a closed box (an oven) and heat the air in the oven to create high-temperature dry heat.

- ✔ **A hot liquid:** You drop the food into a liquid and then heat the liquid. Or you suspend the food over the liquid so that it cooks in the steam escaping from the surface of the boiling liquid.

And that was good enough for centuries of cooks from the caveman to Escoffier and Julia Child. Then whammo! In the waning decades of the 20th century, science delivered a spanking new kitchen heat source, the marvelous microwave oven. A fire (wood, gas, or electric imitation) generates *thermal energy* (heat) that warms and cooks food. A microwave oven generates *electromagnetic energy.*

Microwaves are just plain magical. They sail through glass, paper, and plastic, right into food where they agitate water molecules, which vibrate against each other. The vibration of the water molecules generates more energy (heat) that warms and cooks the food. The dish holding food in a microwave oven generally stays cool because it has so few water molecules.

Fat is yummy. But fat is also a heartburn/reflux trigger. High-fat foods, such as oils and ice cream, are generally regarded as hazardous to your heartburn health. So are foods cooked in ways that add fats. For example, a baked potato is usually okay. Deep-fried French fries are iffy.

To cook your food in ways less likely to set off your heartburn, you need to have a handle on the various techniques. If you don't know the difference between *braise* and *broil,* or *steam* and *stew,* you're not alone. Most people don't. Until, that is, you read through the following list of definitions.

Looking at low-fat cooking methods

Dry low-fat cooking methods, such as roasting, allow fat to drip off food. Wet low-fat cooking methods, such as stewing, allow fat to melt into the liquid, which can then be cooled so that the fat rises to the top and may be lifted off, thus reducing the amount of fat in the finished dish, lowering your risk of heartburn and — incidentally — lowering the calorie count.

- **Baking:** To cook food without liquid in a conventional oven. The word *bake* is used for grain foods such as breads and cakes. For meat, fish, poultry, and sometimes veggies, the word is *roasting.* Baking or roasting reduces fat content because the heat melts the fat, which drips off into the bottom of the pan.

- **Barbecuing:** To cook without liquid over or under an open flame (or electric unit). The food may be marinated before cooking and *basted* (bathed in flavored liquids) during cooking. As with baking/roasting, barbequing reduces fat content because melted fats drip off the barbecued foods.

- **Boiling:** To cook in liquid (water, wine, juice) that has been heated to boiling, 212° F at sea level.

- **Braising:** To cook in a very small amount of liquid (water, wine, juice) in a (usually) covered pot over a low flame. The term is generally applied to meats, sometimes to poultry. *Poaching* is the term used for braising fish, fruits, or vegetables.

- **Broiling:** To cook food directly under an open flame or heating element.

- **Grilling:** To cook directly over hot coals (rather than an open flame, like barbequing) or heating element.

- **Pan-frying:** To cook over high heat with little or no fat, pouring off any fat that accumulates as the food cooks.

- **Pressure-cooking:** To cook in an airtight, covered pan that creates steam under pressure, thus cooking more quickly than ordinary steaming.

- **Steaming:** To cook by placing food on a rack above boiling water.

- **Stewing:** To cook by placing food in moderate amounts of fat-free liquids in a covered pot on top of a heating element or in an oven. Remember to let the liquids cool so you can remove the fat.

Identifying added-fat cooking methods

These techniques add fat to food, lending a crisp tastiness most people find irresistible — but that may set trigger reflux and set your heartburn flaming.

- ✔ **Deep-frying:** To cook by immersing food completely in boiling fat or oil. Think donuts, French fries, and tempura.

- ✔ **Stir-frying:** To cook the Asian way, over high heat, with a small amount of oil. This is more heartburn-friendly than deep-frying, but even a small amount of oil is added fat, which can trigger reflux.

Chapter 7

Reviewing Home Remedies, Alternative Approaches, and Herbal Healers

. . . .

In This Chapter

▶ Checking the value of folk remedies

▶ Figuring out the meaning of *alternative*

▶ Identifying herbal and alternative experts

▶ Listing the virtues of healing herbs

. . . .

*T*hroughout history, ordinary people have often been their own best doctors, especially when treating everyday problems, such as headaches, muscle pains, coughs, colds — and gastric upsets.

Folk medicine books are chock-full of remedies for nausea, constipation, diarrhea, ulcers, and intestinal gas. But mention reflux, and the books become blank slates.

This chapter includes several homespun heartburn remedies to help you soothe the tempest in your tummy. With life's surprises, you're never quite sure when your normally happy innards are likely to rumble, so you will be pleased to discover that some of these home remedies can quiet other gastric upsets as well. If speeding through these few pages may help you alleviate your next unpleasant gastric moment, I say, "Great!"

Grading Granny's Goodies

When you were a kid, and you had a bellyache, gas, nausea, or diarrhea, before Doctor Mom (or Doctor Granny) called the doctor or ran to the drugstore for an over-the-counter (OTC) pill, she probably took pity on your miserable state and prescribed one or more of the following home remedies:

✔ **Ginger ale:** The idea is to replace liquids and minerals lost through vomiting or diarrhea. If the ginger ale actually contained gingerroot, it would qualify as a bona fide antinausea product (more about that later in this chapter).

Some moms and grannies chose to serve cola drinks rather than ginger ale in the mistaken belief that colas contained extract of the coca nut, a sedative that would quiet a jumpy tummy. They weren't quite right. The original formula for cola drinks did contain extracts of the coca plant and the kola nut. The coca extract was a sedative that could indeed calm stomach rumbles. The kola extract, a flavoring.

Modern cola drinks no longer contain the sedative extract, but — unless they're labeled "caffeine free" — they do have lots of caffeine, which means they're definitely not calmer-downers. Better stick to ginger ale.

✔ **Plain crackers or dry toast:** You had to eat something, and these choices provide relatively fat-free, nonirritating calories.

✔ **Hot tea:** Tea has *tannins,* natural compounds that soothe an irritated stomach lining. It also has (shhhh!) caffeine for a nice little lift.

✔ **Applesauce:** Packed with *pectins,* the soluble dietary fiber that counteracts diarrhea well enough to be included in (OTC) antidiarrheal products such as Kao-Pectate.

Clearly Mom and Granny were experts at soothing upset stomachs, but that doesn't mean they were great at fighting reflux. In fact, the homely remedies that may ease gas, nausea, or diarrhea may make reflux worse.

The crackers are okay, but the gas bubbles in ginger ale and the caffeine in tea may loosen the *lower esophageal sphincter* (LES), that pesky trapdoor between your esophagus and stomach. A loosened LES allows acidic stomach liquid to slosh backwards into the esophagus. In others word, reflux. (For more on how reflux happens, turn to Chapter 2.)

If ginger ale, tea, and crackers don't relieve reflux, what exactly do Mom and Granny have to offer?

Neutralizing the burn

Baking soda is plain *sodium bicarbonate,* a natural antacid. Dissolve a teaspoon of the familiar white powder in an 8-ounce glass of water, and presto! you have a solution that neutralizes acid and may temporarily alleviate heartburn due to acid reflux. But following this line of treatment just may have drawbacks.

✔ Dissolving a teaspoon of baking soda in a glass of water releases carbon dioxide, the fizz in the glass. Like the bubbles in ginger ale, the fizz in baking soda can open the LES to enable you to burp up gas.

When the LES opens to allow gas out of your stomach, you feel instant relief from the pressure of "bloat." Unfortunately, opening the LES to burp up gas allows more stomach liquids to slosh back into your esophagus. The baking-soda solution neutralizes some of this acid liquid reflux, but not all. So the burp that relieves bloat may actually prolong your heartburn pain.

✔ Baking soda is high in sodium (see the first word in its chemical name?) so if you're on a low-sodium diet, this remedy probably isn't for you.

✔ Even if sodium is no problem for you, using sodium bicarbonate as your regular antacid may be troublesome. Your body absorbs all the sodium bicarbonate you swallow. Take in too much and you may end up with "clinically significant metabolic alkalosis." *Translation:* A potentially serious imbalance in pH (the acid/base scale described in Chapter 2). Messing up your body's pH isn't good, so take it easy on the baking soda, please.

That list explains why the non-irritating prescription and nonprescription products listed in Chapter 10 pretty much replaced Doctor Mom and Doctor Granny's baking soda burper solution.

Yes, popular antiheartburn products do contain sodium bicarbonate, but not as much per dose as you get by taking your sodium bicarbonate straight from the baking soda box. Besides, if you read the label carefully — which you always do when you take any medicine — you find information about dosing designed to protect you from overdosing.

If you're going to try baking soda, make sure it's baking soda, not baking powder. Why? Get two glasses and I'll show you. First, pour 8 ounces of water into each glass. Now stir a teaspoon of baking soda in one glass and a teaspoon of baking powder in the other. The first foams. The second doesn't. See! Baking soda and baking powder aren't the same product.

Baking soda is plain sodium bicarbonate. Baking powder is a mixture of sodium bicarbonate, cornstarch (to bulk up the powder), calcium phosphate (for firm baked goods), and sodium aluminum sulfate (a flour-bleaching agent). Baking powder makes cakes rise, but it doesn't make you burp or neutralize your stomach acid. For that, you need plain baking soda.

Masticating relief

Mom and Granny's book of heartburn remedies probably doesn't include chewing gum. In fact, the dear women may have mentioned once or twice that chewing gum makes you look like a cow chewing her cud. I wouldn't dream of quarreling with that assessment.

But I can tell you that chewing gum after eating can help neutralize acid reflux and make you feel much better real quick.

Saliva is a mineral-rich natural antacid. Chewing your cud, sorry, chewing your gum stimulates the flow of saliva, which hardens teeth while neutralizing cavity-causing bacterial and food acids. Now you know why many dental researchers recommend your chewing sugarless gum after eating in order to reduce your risk of cavities.

Of course, stomach liquids are also acid. So right about now, you may be asking yourself, "Will chewing gum relieve my heartburn?" Good question. The interesting answer comes from a team of researchers at Britain's Kings College in London who tested chewing gum as a heartburn remedy for 21 volunteers with reflux.

The great pretender

Baking soda (sodium bicarbonate) may not be the ideal heartburn remedy, but it is one of the world's greatest substitutes. Just for starters, you can use it instead of:

✔ **Anti-itch powder:** Make a paste. Dot it on a mosquito bite. Sigh with relief.

✔ **Bath salts:** Add 2 to 3 tablespoons baking soda to a tubful of warm water for a simple mineral water bath. No colors, no fragrances, and no high price.

✔ **General household cleaner:** Two tablespoons dissolved in a quart of warm water do a spiffy job on plaster, tile, and porcelain surfaces.

✔ **Metal polish:** Put a teaspoon of baking soda in a pint of warm soapy water. Scrub stainless steel clean. Ditto for copper and aluminum. But skip the silver: baking soda's too abrasive.

✔ **Oven cleaner:** Sprinkle on some baking soda . . . Scrub. Scrub some more. Scrub even more. Put all your elbow grease behind it, or better yet, give this chore to your teenage son. Eventually the baked-on oven gunk comes off. Yes, it takes longer than caustic oven cleaners, but it doesn't have that awful smell. And it costs a lot less.

✔ **Refrigerator deodorizer:** Open box of baking soda. Put in fridge. Close door. Next.

✔ **Scouring powder:** Forget the kitchen abrasives; rub your pots and pans with baking soda. Neat.

✔ **Toilet bowl cleaner:** Pour a tablespoon of baking soda in the toilet bowl. Scrub sides with toilet brush. Flush. Done.

✔ **Tooth powder:** Make a paste of baking soda and water and brush away stains, even stubborn ones like tea. But get your dentist's okay first: Baking soda may scratch dentures or the soft surface of exposed tooth roots that lack protective super-hard dental enamel.

As Chapter 6 explains, fatty foods loosen the LES and increase the risk of reflux. So for two days, the volunteers ate a high-fat meal and then chewed gum for 30 minutes after one of the fat meals, either on the first or second day. The scientists measured acid levels in each patient's esophagus for two hours after each meal, and then compared the results with and without the chewing gum.

In 2003, the researchers shared the results at *Digestive Disease Week,* an annual whoop-dee-do for *gastroenterologists* (docs who specialize in digestive problems). The data clearly document that chewing away like that proverbial cow can reduce esophageal acidity after eating. Imagine that, Mom! Can you believe it, Granny? Will wonders never cease?

Soothing with a mother's touch

Stress can start your stomach churning, sometimes strongly enough to give you heartburn. When that happens, a gentle touch may ease your stress and offer some relief. As Mom used to say, "Let me kiss it and make it better."

What? You doubt this works? Are you also anti–apple pie? Maybe you had better bookmark this page and turn immediately to Chapter 15, where you can read all about how to cope with stress's negative effects on your body.

Looking for Alternatives

Some people just don't like doctors. When these people get sick, they look for other solutions such as alternative medicine and alternative medicine practitioners. The trouble is that *alternative medicine* is one of those catch phrases people like to toss around without knowing exactly what it means. Not to worry. The explanation of alternative medicine is right here — in the following section.

Defining conventional medicine

Most modern doctors practice *allopathic medicine,* a discipline in which the doctor treats a patient by attempting to induce a condition opposite to what the patient is experiencing. For example, if you have a fever, an allopathic doctor tries to cure you by lowering your body's temperature. If you have an infection, he tries to eliminate the infectious agent(s), almost certainly with antibiotics or antiviral drugs.

Natural versus synthetic

In the world of medical drugs, the line between "natural" and "synthetic" is very fine — and getting finer. Clearly, plants are major sources of effective medicine, such as *vinblastine,* an anticancer compound found in *Vinca rosea* (periwinkle). You can get vinblastine by eating periwinkle flowers, or you can use vinblastine as a synthetic intravenous medicine. Either way, the chemical composition is exactly the same.

So long as you get exactly the same amount of the active ingredient, natural vinblastine and synthetic vinblastine are equally effective. The problem is that establishing the dose of vinblastine in a natural product such as dried or powdered periwinkles is difficult; measuring the units of synthetic vinblastine is a cinch. Ditto for dandelions and furosemide.

Allopathic medicine has won its spurs due to the incredible and thoroughly welcome success of modern "miracle drugs" and vaccines, which have enabled human beings to cure or treat some diseases that were once considered a sure death sentence and eliminate others.

On the other hand, no medical treatment is completely free of side effects. Drugs that cure may also kill. In addition, as medicine becomes more cut and dried, with a pill or a test for every ill, the emotional distance between doctors and patients has widened.

Many patients — and many doctors, too — long for the "good old days," which may not have been so peachy in terms of outcome but did have a certain warmth and friendliness when doctors who had no antibiotics or other modern drugs had to rely on a kindly touch.

Taking a holistic approach

As a result, in the last decades of the 20th century, many patients staged a mini-revolt, turning to alternative forms of medicine in an attempt to revise the relationship between doctors and patients, as well as sometimes to find more comforting — alternative — ways to treat disease.

Alternative medicine is a collection of therapies designed to treat the "whole person," mind (and spirit) as well as body. This kind of medicine is sometimes called *holistic medicine* although spelling that "wholeistic" might be more accurate. There are many different kinds of alternative therapies, but they generally fall into one of three basic approaches:

✔ Therapies such as acupuncture and chiropracty employ physical techniques such as inserting needles at sensitive points on the body or manipulating the spine.

✔ Therapies such as herbal medicine employ "healing substances" such as herbs or food instead of commercial drugs. (For more on herbals and heartburn, see the "Evaluating Herbal Medicines" later in this chapter.)

✔ Therapies such as biofeedback, meditation, and yoga (see Chapter 15) attempt to harness your psychological or intellectual powers to let you control the activities of body systems and functions such as heartbeat once thought to be beyond conscious control.

When an alternative therapy, such as acupuncture, is used together with an ordinary therapy such as pain-relieving drugs, the acupuncture may be described as being *complementary* — that is, added to, the medical treatment.

Evaluating Herbal Medicine

Because many people regularly use herbs and spices to add flavor and zip to their food, they often think of plant seasonings and liquids brewed from plants as totally safe. For the most part, they're right. Yes, some people are sensitive to some plants (for example, if you have hay fever, chamomile tea may make you sneeze), but as a rule, most people use such small amounts of herbs and spices in food that they rarely lead to serious problems.

Using plants as medicine is a different story. To get the benefits of a plant's medically active compounds, you must consume much larger quantities of the herb or spice. In these larger amounts, herbal products may cause some of the problems associated with medical drugs. Medicine-strength herbals may

✔ **Have unpleasant effects:** For example, licorice root, which can coat and soothe a sore throat or heal a gastric ulcer, may cause fluid retention and high blood pressure. (For more on medicine-related problems, check out Chapter 10.)

✔ **Interact with medical drugs and other herbals:** For example, the laxative herb psyllium may delay your body's absorption of medical drugs.

But guess what? Despite these potential problems, herbal products sold in the United States aren't as rigorously regulated as medical drugs.

In the kitchen, you may be accustomed to calling the plants used as seasonings either herbs or spices, but when you're talking remedies, the word is plain and simple: *herbs.* The word for medical products made from plants is *herbals,* which is certainly more graceful than calling some plant remedies herbals and others spice-als.

Viewing herbals and the law

The U.S. Food and Drug Administration (FDA) regulates — no surprise! — food, drugs, and medical devices such as pacemakers. Before the FDA allows a new food, drug, or device to be sold in the United States, the marketer must prove it is safe. For drugs and medical devices, the FDA also says manufactures must prove that the medicine or machine is *efficacious,* a long word for "this product will cure or relieve the condition for which it is prescribed."

Nobody says the system is perfect. Reality dictates that manufacturers can only test a drug on a limited number of people for a limited period of time. So you can bet that some new drugs trigger unexpected, serious, and maybe even life-threatening side effects when used by thousands of people or taken for longer than the testing period. For proof, you need look no further than the drug Phen-Fen. In premarket testing, the diet drug combination appeared to control weight safely. But after the FDA approved and prescribed Phen-Fen for a much wider audience, the FDA quickly realized that taking Phen-Fen could lead to serious, even lethal heart damage, and the FDA pulled the combination from the market.

Unfortunately, the current law prevents the FDA from having similar powers to regulate nutritional supplements — including vitamins, minerals, herbals, and some foods, such as meal-replacement bars and liquids — even though some of these products may potentially be hazardous to a person's health.

Loosening the controls

In 1994, Congress passed and the president signed into law the Dietary Supplement Health and Education Act limiting the FDA's control over dietary supplements, a law that seems intended more to handcuff the FDA rather than to empower the agency to protect Americans. The law

- ✔ Prohibits the FDA from requiring premarket tests to prove supplements are safe and effective.

- ✔ Stops the FDA from limiting the dosage in any dietary supplement.

- ✔ Says the FDA can't halt or restrict sales of a dietary supplement unless the agency has evidence that the product has caused illness or injury when *used according to the directions on the package.* In other words, if you experience a problem after taking slightly more or less of a supplement than directed on the label, the FDA must say, "Sorry, we can't help you."

But you can help the agency help you.

Being a good citizen

Until Congress gives the FDA the tools it needs to ensure the safety of dietary supplements, the agency counts on you to holler when an herbal product is troublesome.

If you experience an adverse effect after using a dietary supplement (you get a headache, you break out in hives, your stomach turns queasy), the FDA wants to hear from you through Medwatch, an information-gathering program that collects and then displays reports on bad news about all kinds of remedies, medical drugs and nutritional supplements alike.

You can dial up the Medwatch hotline at 800-FDA-1088 or log on www.fda.gov/medwatch. Follow the directions to pull up a complaint form or link to related sites. Fill out the form, and zip it off to the FDA. Then give yourself a gold star for good citizenship. Heck, give yourself two.

Looking for expert advice

Herbal products are currently so popular that you can find stories about which one cures what virtually everywhere you turn. The trouble is that the information you get from *The Daily Shout* newspaper, the We Know All About Herbs Web site, or the Buy These Herbs Superstore may not be, shall I say, accurate.

Your better choices for scientifically sound evaluations of herbal products are government agencies or publications that have no financial interest in herbals. I list three of the best in the following sections: The German Commission E, the National Center for Complementary and Alternative Medicine, and *The PDR for Herbal Medicines*.

Getting the goods from Germany

Herbals are serious medicine in Europe. In Germany, for example, the respectful treatment of herbal remedies dates back to the Imperial Decree of 1901, which allowed "botanical drugs" (yes, herbals) to be sold outside of regulated pharmacies.

Time marches on, however, and consumer demand for scientific proof has outstripped the respect for any decree, no matter how imperial. In 1978, the German Minister of Health created Commission E, a regulatory agency charged with evaluating the safety and effectiveness of herbal remedies.

To date, German Commission E has published the results for more than 300 herbs, from A (aconite) to Z (zedoary) in *The Complete German Commission E Monographs*. The book has quickly become a standard reference whose reports characterize specific herbs and/or herbal combinations as either *approved* or *unapproved*.

> ✔ **Approved:** There's reasonable certainty that the herb or herbal combination is safe and effective in a prescribed dose for a specific condition. For example, *angelica root* is an approved herb for treating loss of appetite, intestinal gas, and mild gastric muscle spasms.

> ✔ **Unapproved:** Either there's no proof that the herb is effective or its risks outweigh its benefits. For example, *angelica seeds* and *angelica leaves* are unapproved as a diuretic.

Did you catch the catch in those descriptions? Two different parts of the same plant — in this case, angelica — may have two different ratings based on their effectiveness in treating specific medical conditions.

You can get a copy of the monographs at most bookstores or directly from the publishers, The American Botanical Council in Austin, Texas. If you're really thrifty, you can find them for free by clicking on its Web site at `www.iherb.com/health.html`.

Applying for American aid

The United States' interest in alternative medical therapies was formalized in 1992 with the creation of the National Center for Complementary and Alternative Medicine (NCCAM). By law, NCCAM is charged with overseeing research on alternative therapies, including herbal medicine.

NCCAM is one of 27 institutes and centers at the National Institutes of Health (NIH), a division of the U.S. Department of Health and Human Services (HHS). What's that mean exactly? Stick close to me here; tracking your way through a government organization chart can get really twisty.

> ✔ **Level One:** First is the U.S. Department of Health and Human Services (HHS), an enormous agency charged with setting the rules for health and human services.

> ✔ **Level Two:** HHS oversees eight agencies, one of which is the Public Health Service (PHS).

> ✔ **Level Three:** PHS is in charge of the National Institutes of Health (NIH), a conglomeration of 27 institutes and centers, each devoted to a specific aspect of medicine.

> ✔ **Level Four:** And finally, you find NCCAM, one of the 27 NIH institutes and centers.

NCCAM has a straightforward mission to

> ✔ Determine the safety and effectiveness of complementary and alternative medicine (CAM) therapies and products

> ✔ Disseminate information to the public and medical professionals on which CAM therapies and products work, which don't, and why

> ✔ Integrate proven CAM therapies and products into conventional medicine, dentistry, and nursing

✔ Support rigorous research on CAM

✔ Train researchers in CAM

NCCAM's Web site (`http://nccam.nih.gov`) is packed to the virtual rafters with information about alternative treatments plus links to more than 220,000, yes, 220,000, scientific citations related to complementary and alternative medicine. Are you really hipped on alternative therapies? Sign up for the NCCAM newsletter online or by snail mail.

To contact NCCAM, you can phone 888-644-6226 or 301-519-3153; TTY (for deaf or hard-of-hearing callers) 866-464-3615. Or you can e-mail `info@nccam.nih.gov`. You can also send snail mail to NCCAM Clearinghouse, P.O. Box 7923, Gaithersburg, MD 20898-7923. To fax the NCCAM, use 866-464-3616 or to use the fax-on-demand service, dial 888-644-6226.

The Web site enables you to enter the NCCAM data banks in search of info on herbs or herbals. Simply type the name of an herb into the search bar on the home page to come up with what's known (and not known) about its medical value. Be warned, though: When I typed "heartburn", "reflux", and "GERD" into the NCCAM Web site search engine, it flunked the test. Can you believe it? No entries at all!

For more specific information on herbal products in U.S. stores, you may want to flip through a copy of *The PDR for Herbal Medicines* (Medical Economics). (The initials PDR stand for the old familiar Physicians' Desk Reference.) The PDR's herbal profiles are up-to-date, complete with dosage and safety information, evaluation of their effectiveness, a guide to adverse effects and interactions, news about clinical trials, and — best of all — notes on specific brand-name products, including those available in your home town.

Tea time tea terms

Herbals are often served as warm drinks called teas, but properly speaking, the word *tea* applies only to the beverage made from the leaves of the tea plant, *Camellia sinensis*.

Pour boiling water over chopped leaves, let the mixture sit in the cup or teapot for a few minutes before serving, and what you have is an *infusion,* sometimes known as a *tisane.*

If you pour boiling water over herbs and continue to heat the mixture on the stove or over a small brazier, the result is a *decoction.* As a general rule, an infusion is made from the soft parts of a plant, such as leaves, while a decoction is made from harder plant parts such as seeds and roots.

Classifying stomach-friendly herbals

All the reliable guides classify herbs and herbal products according to their therapeutic function. Herbals that alleviate gastric unpleasantries, such as nausea, gas, constipation, and diarrhea, generally fall into one of the following categories:

- **Antiemetics:** They relieve nausea and reduce the incidence of vomiting. Ginger root is an antiemetic herb.

- **Antispasmodics:** They relax intestinal muscles, relieving painful muscle spasms. Anise seed and dill seed are antispasmodic herbs.

- **Appetite stimulants:** They trigger the flow of gastric juices and set off hunger pangs. Angelica root is an appetite-stimulant herb.

- **Carminatives:** They prevent the formation of intestinal gas or help expel it from your body. Caraway and fennel are carminative herbs.

- **Demulcents:** They create a soothing protective layer over sensitive mucous membranes, such as the lining of your mouth and throat. Licorice root is a demulcent herb.

- **Laxatives:** They help bulk up stool and increase peristalsis. Flaxseed and senna are laxative herbs.

- **Saliva stimulants:** They increase the secretion of saliva. Gentian root stimulates saliva secretion.

The German Commission E rates the herbals listed in Table 7-1 as "approved" for treating gastric upset. Look over this list carefully. See anything that may relieve heartburn? The correct response would definitely be a *very* cautious *maybe* for gentian root, ginger, licorice, and marshmallow.

Gentian and ginger stimulate the flow of saliva, the natural antacid that may help wash irritating stomach acid out of your esophagus. Licorice and marshmallow are demulcents that can lay down a protective coating on the mucous membranes lining your digestive tract. In fact, glycyrrhizia (pronounced gli-ci-*ri*-zee-ah), the active ingredient in licorice root, was once an ingredient in conventional medications used to heal ulcers.

So why be so cautious about calling these heartburn healers? Because the truth is that in a real stomach (as opposed to the page of even the most reliable herbal guide) no herbal product is likely to relieve reflux as effectively as a conventional medicine.

Herbals are medicine-strength products. Never use one without checking with your doctor first, particularly if you're being treated for a chronic medical condition such as diabetes, arthritis, or asthma. And, of course, a smart cookie like you always reads all those important directions printed in teensy "mouse type" on the label.

Table 7-1	Herbal Help for an Upset Stomach	
Herb (Part Used)	**Functions**	**Possible Unpleasant Effects**
Aloe (leaves, latex)	Laxative	Cramps; loss of important minerals, including potassium; interacts with drugs used to treat irregular heartbeat; makes the heart medication digitalis stronger
Angelica (root)	Antispasmodic, appetite stimulant, carminative	Handling the plant may cause dermatitis
Anise (seed)	Antispasmodic	Skin, respiratory, and gastrointestinal allergic reactions
Caraway (seed)	Antispasmodic, carminative	**
Chamomile (flowers)	Antispasmodic	Respiratory allergic reactions
Cinnamon (bark)	Antispasmodic, carminative	Allergic irritation to skin and mucous membranes
Cloves (buds)	Antispasmodic	Irritation of mucous membrane lining mouth, throat, stomach
Coriander (seed)	Appetite stimulant; soothes upset stomach	**
Dandelion (leaves, stems)	Appetite stimulant	Allergic reactions; if you have gallstones, check with your doctor before using dandelions
Dill (seed)	Antispasmodic	**
Fennel (seed)	Antispasmodic,* carminative	Skin, respiratory allergic reactions
Flaxseed (seed)	Laxative	No side effects if taken as directed with liquids

(continued)

Table 7-1 *(continued)*

Herb (Part Used)	Functions	Possible Unpleasant Effects
Gentian (root)	Appetite stimulant, carminative, saliva stimulant	Headache (rare)
Ginger (root)	Antiemetic, saliva stimulant	Increases strength of "blood thinners" such as warfarin; if you have gallstones, check with doctor before using ginger
Horehound	Appetite stimulant, carminative	**
Licorice	Demulcent	**
Marshmallow	Demulcent	**
Peppermint (leaf)	Antispasmodic	If you have gallstones, check with doctor before using peppermint
Psyllium (seed)	Laxative	Allergic reactions
Rosemary (leaf)	Antispasmodic	**
Senna (leaf, pod)	Laxative	Cramps; potassium deficiency; strengthens heart medication digitalis; interacts with drugs used to treat irregular heartbeat
Star anise (seed)	Antispasmodic	**

*Low concentrations increase peristalsis, the muscle contractions that move food through your intestinal tract.
** No unpleasant effects noted in the German Commission E report.
Source: Blumenthal, et al., The Complete German Commission E Monographs *(American Botanical Council) 1998.*

Shopping smart

The last word — okay, the last two words — on herbal remedies is/are: Shop smart.

Look for a fresh product from a reputable manufacturer that will last long enough to give you the best bang for the buck. Before you plunk down good money for an herbal remedy, check out the checklist in Table 7-2. Answer each question. Lots of "Yes" answers tell you the product you're looking at is probably right for you. Ready? Set. Check!

Table 7-2 Picking a Product		
Ask Yourself This Question	*Yes*	*No*
Does the product have a respected brand name?	❏	❏
Are the letters USP (for U.S. Pharmacopoeia, a reputable testing organization) on the label?	❏	❏
Is the package tamper-proof and sealed?	❏	❏
Is the expiration date far enough in the future so you can use the herbal before it expires?	❏	❏
Is the herbal stored safely? (For example, is a product that requires refrigeration kept in the store's fridge?)	❏	❏
Is the product the most effective form of the herb (real herbs — leaves, stems, seeds — generally rate higher than capsules and pills)?	❏	❏
Are you sensitive to anything on the ingredient list?	❏	❏
Are the label claims too good to be true?	❏	❏
Did your doctor say it's okay to use this herbal?	❏	❏

Don't try this at home

Do you hate taking heartburn medicine? Compare your medicine to the 19th-century homemade heartburn herbal remedy:

✔ 3 drams sulphite of soda

✔ 3 drams sal volatile

✔ 2 drams tincture of ginger

✔ 8 oz infusion of quassia

Translation: A dram is ⅛ ounce. Sulphite of soda is sort of like sodium bicarbonate. Sal volatile is smelling salts, a mixture of alcohol, ammonia, and fragrant oils whose sharp odor revived folks who had fainted. Quassia is a bitter tonic, once used in enemas.

Linking Other Alternative Approaches to Heartburn/Reflux

Overall, alternative medicine doesn't play a large part in treating heartburn/reflux. In fact, it pains me to point out that when I typed *heartburn,* then *reflux,* then *GERD,* and finally *gastrointestinal reflux disease* into the NCCAM search bar, I got back zero, zip, zilch. Hey, maybe it was a bad day.

But I'm relieved to note that the World Health Organization (WHO) does recommend acupuncture as an effective treatment for lots of different conditions, including two of interest to people with heartburn: esophageal spasms and a stomach that churns out too much acid.

Want to know more about acupuncture? A good source is the American Academy of Medical Acupuncture (AAMA), founded in 1987 by physicians who had graduated from the Medical Acupuncture for Physicians Training Program at the UCLA School of Medicine. The AAMA is the sole physician-only professional acupuncture society in North America accepting members from a diversity of training backgrounds. You can reach them at www.medicalacupuncture.org.

Several alternative stress-reduction techniques such as biofeedback may also help some people relieve their heartburn, but that's a subject for Chapter 15, which details the connection between stress and reflux — and suggests ways in which to deal with your stress.

Part III
Treating Your Middle

The 5th Wave   By Rich Tennant

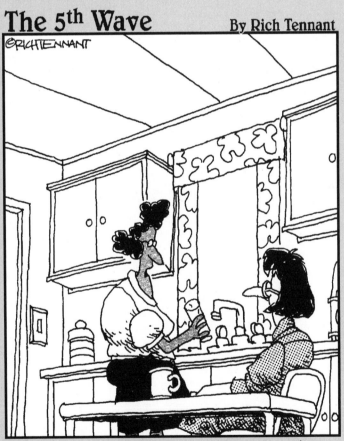

"Heartburn? I like the medication that shows 2 people in a rowboat having a picnic, but Cliff likes the one with 2 people on Roman holiday eating lasagne."

In this part . . .

Help! You're looking for a way to soothe your heartburn pain. This part tells you how to find a doctor,
lists the test she may prescribe, and tells you everything you need to know about medicines that relieve
heartburn — and those meds that may make it worse.
Finally, you can find out about surgery, the last-resort
heartburn treatment.

Chapter 8

Finding the Right Doctor

· ·

In This Chapter

▶ Determining when you need medical assistance

▶ Naming the doctors who treat heartburn

▶ Visiting the doctor with a list in hand

· ·

*I*f you already have both a primary care physician (PCP) and a gastroenterologist, and you're satisfied with both, you can skip this chapter. On the
other hand, if you haven't yet set up your heartburn/reflux medical team or if
you have questions about the doctors you're dealing with now, sit down and
take a look.

What you find in this chapter can help you decide whether you need medical
help, which doctors provide it, how to find a doctor in your neighborhood,
and — best of all — how to evaluate the quality of any doctors to whom you
choose to deliver your precious bod. I even help you prepare to walk into the
gastro doc's office for the first time.

Finally, don't forget to read the sidebar on medical directives, the "second
wills" which give you the opportunity to enforce your medical decisions under
all circumstances, even the most dire, a nervous-making but necessary step.

Deciding When to See the Doctor

For people with heartburn, four simple reasons say, "Time to seek professional help."

- ✔ **Reason No. 1:** Your heartburn happens more than once a week, maybe
  even every day.

- ✔ **Reason No. 2:** Changing your diet or rearranging your meal schedule as
  suggested in Chapter 6 hasn't doused the fire.

✔ **Reason No. 3:** Simple home remedies like those in Chapter 7 haven't relieved the pain for long, and neither have the nonprescription medicines listed in Chapter 10.

✔ **Reason No. 4:** Your heartburn is teamed with other unpleasant symptoms, such as a persistent cough, postnasal drip, asthma, constipation, diarrhea, or any of the health-related risk factors found in Chapter 4.

Face it. These events are your body's way of sending you a clear message: "Take me to the doctor, please."

If you experience a gastrointestinal emergency, such as coughing up blood, ignore all rules. Run, don't walk to the nearest emergency room. If you cough up more than a splotch of blood on a tissue, dial 911 for assistance. Right away. This isn't a time to procrastinate.

Sorting Through the Heartburn Specialists

Once upon a time, a person had one kindly doctor who did everything from delivering babies to yanking out appendices, treating chronic diseases, running medical tests, and — sorry about this — closing the patient's eyes at The End.

Today, the incredible explosion in medical information, knowledge, and technique makes it impossible for any one doctor, no matter how smart and caring, to keep up with advances in multiple disciplines. So

✔ Babies arrive via the services of an obstetrician/gynecologist, a family physician, or a licensed midwife.

✔ Surgeons trained to deal with specific organs and systems remove, repair, or replace the appendix — and various other body parts.

✔ Cardiologists, rheumatologists, and whole bunches of other *-ists* treat individual chronic illnesses.

✔ Lab techs perform lab tests.

✔ As for the aforementioned The End, you can't believe how many different doctors have a hand in seeing you through. (If you want to check out more about what you need to do to prepare, check out the sidebar "Where there's a will, there's another will" in this chapter.)

Given the confusing plethora of medical personnel, even people not enrolled in a health maintenance organization (HMO) have come to accept the medical delivery system these groups pioneered in which one doctor — your PCP — acts as a kind of conductor, coordinating the players in your very own personal medical band.

But just who are the heartburn players the PCP directs? The list varies with the medical condition, but for people with heartburn/reflux, the ensemble may include these folks (in likely order of their appearance in your medical life after you leave the PCP):

- **Gastroenterologist:** A physician who specializes in diseases of the digestive tract. Gastroenterologists are the doctors best equipped to order the tests required to diagnose and evaluate your heartburn/reflux (see Chapter 9 for more on the diagnostic tests for heartburn).

- **Endoscopist:** A physician (usually, but not always, a gastroenterologist) trained in the use of an *endoscope,* a slim tube that accommodates a small TV camera, which enables the doctor to peer into the esophagus in order to evaluate the condition of the esophageal lining, a valuable clue to your reflux's severity.

- **Radiologist:** A doctor who specializes in the use of imaging techniques, such as X-rays, CT scans, ultrasound, and magnetic resonance imaging (MRI), to diagnose or treat disease. For people with heartburn, the radiologist is the person who performs tests such as the barium swallow used to identify irregularities in the esophagus.

- **Gastroenterological surgeon:** The doctor who operates on the organs of the digestive system. (Do you want to know more about heartburn surgery? See Chapter 12.)

- **Technician:** An increasingly important member of the medical team who's skilled in running medical tests. The technician isn't a medical doctor; he works under the direction of your doctor, radiologist, or surgeon.

Each of these people may play a role in deciding whether you have reflux and if so, how to treat it. Your task is to pick the right person for the job.

Choosing a Doctor

Most people wouldn't hire a plumber without first checking references and licensing, but we often blithely skip off to a new doctor without looking for similar assurances.

I'm going to assume that you've known your PCP for some time. Your first reference for a gastro specialist is most likely to be your PCP. The fact that your trusted PCP recommended the specialist should be reassuring. But you'll also want to do some checking on your own before you walk in the office door. Your PCP's referral doesn't have to be the last word. Except in life-and-death emergencies (an unlikely situation when the complaint is heartburn), you're smart to check out your doctor before she gets to check you out.

Start by finding answers to the basic questions: Does the doctor practice close to your home? Is she associated with a hospital near you? And — this is a tricky one — have any of your friends been to see her, and do they have an opinion? (I said it was tricky.)

Then take time to conduct some further research. The following sections provide some advice. Armed with this info, make an appointment — or have your PCP make one for you. (Check out the "Going to the Doctor with Your History in Hand" section later in this chapter to find out how you can make that first trip to the gastro specialist a productive one.)

Basic credentials

First you want to know if your doctor is qualified to poke and prod the body parts that bother you. In other words, does he have the credentials I need to provide the medical answers I require? One way to be sure is to check out whether he is *board certified*.

The American Board of Medical Specialties (ABMS) and the American Medical Association (AMA) recognize 24 specialty boards, many with their own subspecialties. A doctor who meets the training requirements of a board and passes his examination is said to be *board certified*.

Gastroenterology is a subspecialty of the American Board of Internal Medicine. To be certified as a gastroenterologist, an aspiring doctor must first be certified as an internal medicine specialist, which means he must (in this order):

- ✔ Graduate from medical school
- ✔ Have a license to practice medicine
- ✔ Complete several years of full-time training (residency) in his field of specialization
- ✔ Obtain a recommendation from his superior
- ✔ Pass a written examination given by the specialty board

Wait! That's just the first step. To make it all the way to gastroenterologist, the doctor must

✔ Go through three years of accredited training (including 18 months working with patients) in the diagnosis and management of a broad spectrum of gastroenterological diseases.

✔ Become proficient in the following techniques:

- Colonoscopy, including biopsy and polypectomy

- Diagnostic upper gastrointestinal endoscopy

- Esophageal dilation

- Liver biopsy

- Proctoscopy and/or flexible sigmoidoscopy

- Therapeutic upper and lower gastrointestinal endoscopy

Having completed these tasks, he gets his name listed in *The Official ABMS Directory of Board Certified Medical Specialists,* so his patients — and his parents — can see it in black and white. You can check out the directory on the ABMS Web site (www.abms.org) or ask about a prospective doc on the toll-free line: 800-ASK-ABMS (800-275-2267). The newly minted gastroenterologist also gets a certificate to hang on his wall.

Endoscopists, gastroenterological surgeons, and radiologists all go through similarly rigorous training, the difference being that after finishing medical school

✔ Endoscopists emphasize training in endoscopic techniques.

✔ Gastroenterological surgeons are trained in surgery and may also have some training in gastroenterology and endoscopy.

✔ Radiologists study radiological techniques and tests.

Professional associations

After you know what to look for, the question is where to look? If you're a member of a healthcare group such as an HMO, you already have a handy-dandy catalog of qualified doctors.

If you don't have a list handy, medical professional associations are a simple way to look for a specialist in your area. When you're talkin' heartburn/reflux, the relevant groups are

✔ The American College of Gastroenterology (www.acg.gi.org)

✔ American College of Radiology (www.acr.org)

✔ American Gastroenterological Association (www.gastro.org)

✔ American Society for Gastrointestinal Endoscopy (www.asge.org)

Each of these Web sites has a search function. The radiology folks also have a search engine for accredited imaging facilities by zip code.

State medical societies

Yet another way to check up on credentials or search for a local specialist is your state medical society. For a quick click, the AMA has a Web site with links to 43 states and the District of Columbia at www.ama-assn.org/ama/pub/category/7630.html.

No, I don't know why the AMA left seven states off its list, but this *For Dummies* book certainly isn't going to leave you six states short of a complete list. Table 8-1 has the Web sites for 49, count 'em, 49 states plus the District. What state is missing? Alaska, which doesn't have a Web site for its medical society, but does have an e-mail address, which I include on the chart.

Click carefully. Not all the Web addresses in Table 8-1 start with www.

Table 8-1		Clicking with the States	
State	*Medical Society Web Site*	*State*	*Medical Society Web Site*
Alabama	www.masalink.org	Connecticut	www.csms.org
Alaska *	asma@alaska.net	Delaware	www.medsocdel.org
Arizona	www.azmedassn.	District of Columbia	www.msdc.org
Arkansas	www.arkmed.org	Florida	www.fmaonline.org
California	www.cmanet.org	Georgia	www.mag.org
Colorado	www.cms.org	Hawaii	www.hmaonline.net

State	Medical Society Web Site	State	Medical Society Web Site
Idaho	www.idmed.org	New York	http://mssny.org
Illinois	www.isms.org	North Carolina	www.ncmedsoc.org
Indiana	www.ismanet.org	North Dakota	http://ndmed.org
Iowa	www.iowamedical.org	Ohio	www.osma.org
Kansas	www.kmsonline.org	Oklahoma	http://osmaonline.org
Kentucky	www.kyma.org	Oregon	www.theoma.org
Louisiana	www.lsms.org	Pennsylvania	www.pamedsoc.org
Maine	www.mainemed.com	Rhode Island	www.rimed.org
Maryland	www.medchi.org	South Carolina	www.scmanet.org
Massachusetts	www.massmed.org	South Dakota	www.sdsma.org
Michigan	www.msms.org	Tennessee	www.medwire.org
Minnesota	www.mnmed.org	Texas	www.texmed.org
Mississippi	www.msmaonline.com	Utah	www.utahmed.org
Missouri	www.msma.org	Vermont	www.vtmd.org
Montana	www.mmaoffice.com	Virginia	www.msv.org
Nebraska	www.nebmed.org	Washington	www.wsma.org
Nevada	www.nsmadocs.org	West Virginia	www.wvsma.com
New Hampshire	www.nhms.org	Wisconsin	www.wisconsinmedicalsociety.org
New Jersey	www.msnj.org	Wyoming	www.wyomed.org
New Mexico	www.nmms.org		

*This is an e-mail address, not a Web site.

Diagnosing doctor roles

Hollywood and TV have a rich history of medical movies, usually starring doctors so handsome and compassionate you can see the halo floating above their well-coiffed heads. Can you match the stars with their famous roles? Give it a try, secure in the knowledge that none of these heroes would ever make any Bad Doc List.

Movie	Movie Star
1. *Doc Hollywood* (1991)	a. Spencer Tracy
2. *The Doctor* (1991)	b. Eddie Murphy
3. *Doctor in the House* (1954)	c. Michael J. Fox
4. *Doctor Doolittle* (1967)	d. Jean Hersholt
5. *Doctor Doolittle* (1998)	e. Rex Harrison
6. *Doctor Zhivago* (1965)	f. Omar Sharif
7. *Meet Dr. Christian* (1939)	g. Dirk Bogard
8. *Dr. Cyclops* (1940)	h. Lew Ayres
9. *Dr. Jekyll and Mr. Hyde* (1941)	i. Albert Dekker
10. *Calling Dr. Kildare* (1939)	j. William Hurt
11. *Dr. Jekyll and Mr. Hyde* (1931)	k. Frederic March

Answers: 1. c, 2. j, 3. g, 4. e, 5. b, 6. f, 7. d, 8. i, 9. a, 10. h, 11. k

State health departments

This statement is unpleasant but true: Not every doctor is a good guy or gal — or even a competent professional. As a result, some patients have frustrating experiences, some are injured, and some sadly end up in legal tangles attempting to (in the legal phrase) "make themselves whole" (get compensated for the damage done to them).

Doctors are licensed by the states in which they practice. In recent years, some state health departments have begun to list malpractice information for individual doctors in the doctors' files on each state's Web site. One excellent example is the New York Department of Health Web site (www.health.state.ny.us), which has a file for every doctor in the state. The file — a medical consumer's dream — shows each doctor's

✔ Education

✔ Hospital affiliation

- ✔ Malpractice judgment and/or settlements
- ✔ Professional activities
- ✔ Publications
- ✔ Specialty

Unfortunately, there's no national database similar to what's provided by New York (and several other consumer-friendly state governments). All the state health departments list the doctors licensed to practice in the state, but not all list every little detail provided in a complete directory such as New York's. The most likely information to be missing is — you guessed — material relating to malpractice. If your state doesn't list this information, you'll find getting the data someplace else difficult if not impossible. In which case, your job as an intelligent medical consumer is to talk to your local politicians and demand that they make the stats available.

Going to the Doctor with Your History in Hand

Walking into a doctor's office often seems to produce a kind of "patient's amnesia." You forget why you're upset, you forget your symptoms, you forget what meds you're taking . . . heck, you may even forget your name if it weren't written right there on the chart in the doctor's hand.

To forestall forgetting, make a list and bring it to your first appointment with the specialist. Make two. Heck, make three. No, make five.

- ✔ **Medical history:** List the illnesses you've had and the medicines and nutritional supplements you've taken.

- ✔ **Family history:** List examples of similar problems in your family. For example, if you have heartburn after eating hot dogs and your mother does, too, tell him that, too.

- ✔ **Current complaint:** Write down what currently ails you and the symptoms that brought you up the medical ladder. For example, your heartburn started out as a twinge after those hot dogs once in a while and then escalated to a burning pain in the middle after every meal. In addition, you're slightly nauseated. And every so often, the whole thing gives you a headache.

- ✔ **Actions taken to date:** Record what you've done so far to ease your problem. For example, you gave up hot dogs, you tried over-the-counter antacids, and then your PCP suggested you try over-the-counter H2-blockers and proton pump inhibitors (read all about it in Chapter 10), but none of them put out the fire in the center of your chest.

✔ **Current medicines:** Make a list of every single medical product that passes your lips each day — not just your heartburn medicines, but any drug you're taking for a current condition. And don't forget to include vitamins and minerals.

Physical exams, in general are truly annoying. You gotta get undressed in front of a stranger who then pokes about your body looking for heaven knows what while muttering, "h'mmmmmm," at strategic intervals. But you'd be amazed at what your doctor can find out by poking and prodding. Sometimes the surprise is good (you have gas, not reflux), sometimes it's useful (sorry, you have reflux).

In addition to an exam, people with heartburn may also undergo a number of diagnostic tests listed in Chapter 9 — unless the problem really is gas, and you're excused from further poking.

Where there's a will, there's another will

Congratulations. The whole thing gave you goose bumps, but you did it anyway. You wrote a will divvying up your assets — your i-Pod to your brother, your laptop to your sister, your signed Yankees cap to your dad, and Fluffy the cat to your mom (who else can you trust with such a sensitive concern?). Then you had the will witnessed and notarized, and stuck it away in your desk with a sigh of relief. Well, hold that sigh. You have one more goose-bump task to go, creating a *medical directive.*

In 1990, the U.S. Congress passed the Patient Self-Determination Act, a law giving all competent Americans older than 18 the right to decide what medical treatment to accept at the end of life. The law says every hospital or nursing home that receives federal funds must tell you about your options when you enter. But by the time you get to the hospital or nursing home you may be unconscious or otherwise unable to make important decisions. Better to have your intentions spelled out in advance via a medical directive, a two-part document that goes into effect immediately if you are so sick or badly injured that you can't express your wishes.

The first part of your medical directive is your *declaration* (what many people call a *living will*),

a statement of what kinds of medical care you do and don't want. For example, if your brain is no longer functioning and there is no reasonable hope of your recovering, do you want to be kept alive on machines that breathe for you? How do you feel about feeding tubes?

The second part of your medical directive is a *durable power of attorney for healthcare,* a document that names a trusted relative, friend, or acquaintance to make decisions regarding your medical treatment when you're incapacitated.

The scenario sounds scary (breathing machines? feeding tubes?), but a medical directive is actually an antiscare device to keep medical decisions in the hands of people you know and trust rather than tossing them off to people who've never met you.

The laws regarding medical directives differ from state to state, so you must consult a lawyer — or your state medical society — for the particulars. Do it. Write it. Sign it. And make lots of copies. One for your doctor, one for your brother, one for your sister, one for mom and dad, one for Fluffy . . . and then go out and live your life. Free of goose bumps.

Chapter 9

Examining Your Esophagus and Testing Your Tummy

. . . .

In This Chapter
▶ Selecting patients who qualify for testing
▶ Describing the tests for GERD
▶ Listing tests for esophageal damage

. . . .

*I*f simply thinking about medical tests sends shivers up and down your spine, you may want to skip this chapter. Or you could take a deep breath and plunge into this catalog of diagnostic procedures.

The tests in this chapter are ones your doctor can order up to figure what's giving you that pain in the middle, pinpoint the problem's effects on your esophagus, and recommend treatment to make you feel ever so much better.

Sounds like a pretty good return on a few minutes of squirmy reading, don't you think?

Picking Potential Patients

When you check in for your annual checkup, do you tuck a checklist into your purse or pocket to remind you to ask your doctor for these tests?

 ✔ Cholesterol check

 ✔ Complete blood count (CBC)

 ✔ Mammogram (for women)

 ✔ Prostate specific antigen (PSA; the test for prostate cancer for men)

If reading this list makes you wince (not to mention thinking about all the countless other exams that record the workings of every single cell in your healthy little body), then contemplating tests that may be required to diagnose the pain in your middle may send you on to Panic Land. But cancel your ticket.

Even in the Age of Medical Miracles, when every little symptom has a test of its own, not every case of heartburn requires testing. If your heartburn responds to changes in your diet or to antacids and antireflux meds, the good news is that you can pretty much forget about delivering your esophagus for expert evaluation.

On the other hand, your doctor may suggest testing if

- ✔ You've had the pain for years but aren't sure your heartburn comes from gastroesophageal reflux disease (GERD).

- ✔ Your symptoms don't respond to dietary changes, such as the ones I suggest in Chapter 6, or to potent antireflux meds, such as proton pump inhibitors (PPIs), one class of drugs described in Chapter 10.

- ✔ You develop signs of serious illness, such as unexplained weight loss or difficulty in swallowing, or a genuine emergency, such as esophageal bleeding.

- ✔ You're scheduled for heartburn surgery.

If you fit into one of these categories, prepare to have your acidity measured, your muscles tested, your stomach observed, and your esophagus examined — after your doctor rules out other possible causes for these symptoms. For example, because the pain of reflux-related heartburn can be so similar to the pain of heart disease, your doctor may order an electrocardiogram to be sure the problem isn't your heart.

As you read through the following list of tests, two questions may come to mind: Where will my test be done and what kind of anesthesia will I be given? These questions are sensible. Unfortunately, I don't have an absolute, every time, no-matter-what answer. A fluoroscopic exam, for example, may be done at a hospital radiology department or at a free-standing (not-in-a-hospital) site run by a group of radiologists. An endoscopy may be done in a doctor's office (which may or may not be in a hospital) or in a hospital surgical unit. The site is generally up to your doctor. Sometimes your insurance coverage or rules specific to your state may also play a role. As for anesthesia, your doctor determines that based on the test and perhaps your own physical condition.

Assessing Your Acidity

Unless you're experiencing a medical emergency — spitting up blood, for example — your doctor is likely to begin with the simplest test to make sure the pain in your middle is really heartburn. In other words, he wants to know if the environment in your esophagus is acidic enough to be the result of reflux.

The diagnostic gold standards for assessing your acidity are

✔ A test that measures how sensitive your esophagus is to acid reflux

✔ A test that measures how acidic the liquid in your esophagus really is

And luckily, these tests are readily available.

Bernstein test (acid perfusion test)

The *Bernstein test,* named for American internist Lionel Bernstein who created it, *perfuses* (sprinkles or washes) a liquid over the lining of your esophagus to measure the sensitivity of your esophageal lining to two different liquids — a salt (saline) solution and a weakly acid solution.

Preparing for this test

Don't consume any food or beverages for at least 12 hours before the test. Also avoid any antacid or antireflux medicine for at least 24 hours before the test.

Taking this test

The doctor, nurse, or technician running this test inserts a thin tube into your nose and down into your esophagus, while explaining how you can quell the normal gag reflex that may prevent the tube from entering smoothly. When the tube is in place, he drips some ordinary saline (saltwater) solution through and asks if it hurts. Next, he drips a weak acid solution through the tube and, once again, asks how you feel.

No, you can't cheat by finding out the answers in advance. To make sure the test is accurate, the doctor may reverse the order, giving you acid first and saltwater second. After you've been exposed to both solutions and the doctor has noted your responses, he withdraws the tube, and you're done.

Evaluating the results

And here are your results:

✔ No pain with either solution? Congratulations. The lining of your esophagus is smooth and healthy.

✔ Did you have pain with the acid solution but not with the saline solution? Your heartburn is probably due to acid reflux.

✔ Did you have pain with both solutions? Your doctor may want to look further to find the cause of your discomfort.

Ambulatory 24-hour pH monitoring

As Chapter 2 explains, *pH* is the term used to describe the acidity of a water-based solution, such as the reflux in your esophagus. For reasons known only to Søren Peter Lauritz Sørensen, the Swedish chemist who created pH, the more acid the solution, the lower its number on the pH scale. For example:

- ✔ pH of hydrochloric acid equals 1.
- ✔ pH of lemon juice and stomach juices equals 2.
- ✔ pH of soft drinks and vinegar equals 3.

Gastroenterologists generally regard an esophageal pH level of 4 — about the pH of tomato juice — as characteristic of GERD. To measure the acidity of your esophageal environment, this test

- ✔ Determines the pH of the reflux in your esophagus
- ✔ Keeps track of how long the reflux liquids linger in your esophagus
- ✔ Records the number of times you experience acid reflux in one 24-hour period

Ambulatory 24-hour pH monitoring — a test that runs a full day while you are *ambling,* sorry, walking around — takes longer and is more annoying than the Bernstein test, but it gives your doctor a more accurate record of the factors that confirm a diagnosis of GERD.

Preparing for this test

Don't consume any food and liquids for 12 hours before the test. Also avoid antacids, antireflux medicines, alcohol, antidepressants, antihistamines, anti-Parkinson drugs, antispasmodics, muscle relaxants, and steroid drugs for 24 hours before the test, unless your doctor has instructed you otherwise.

Actually, asking your doctor about how he wants you to handle your usual medications ahead of time is a good move. That way, you're both on the same page.

Taking this test

The doctor or medical technician running the test inserts a very fine tube into your nose, down your throat, and into your esophagus. The tube, which stays in place for 24 hours, has a teensy electronic probe at the end that relays data to a recorder that you carry in your pocket to register the acidity in your esophagus during that 24-hour period. Though it sounds horrible, the test doesn't interfere with your normal daily activity. And no, the tube can't slip down into your body and get lost in your stomach. Well, that's a relief!

Some gee-whiz gastro guys have come up with a new 48-hour esophageal acidity test using a small, wireless capsule inserted through a tube and tacked onto the esophagus wall just above the stomach's entrance. After the device is in place, the doctor or medical technician removes the tube and the capsule begins to send acidity info to a recorder you wear at your waist. After the study, the data are sent to a computer and analyzed. The capsule falls off within five days and makes it way out of your digestive tract in the usual manner.

The benefit of the capsule test is obvious: No unsightly, uncomfortable tube hanging from your nose. The drawbacks:

- ✔ Its expense
- ✔ The possibility that the capsule will drop off prematurely or fail to transmit data

As a result, this capsule test isn't yet the default mode. But stay tuned. You never know.

Evaluating the results

The possible outcomes are

- ✔ If your data show frequent reflux and high acidity, your doctor assumes you have GERD.
- ✔ If you're already taking medicine for your heartburn, but this test shows that you still have lots of acid in your esophagus, your doctor can use the results to adjust the dosage or change the medicine to give you more-effective relief.
- ✔ If you don't have a high level of acidity, you may not have GERD, which means your doctor must look for other causes for your pain.

Your doctor may also use this test to evaluate patients scheduled for heartburn surgery (see Chapter 12) to be certain that the patients actually have the abnormal levels of highly acid reflux that qualify them for the procedures.

Measuring Your Muscle Strength

Two types of muscles play an important role in protecting you from reflux:

> ✔ **The muscles in the esophageal walls:** These muscles exert rhythmic contractions called *peristalsis,* which move food down to your stomach.
>
> ✔ **The lower esophageal sphincter (LES):** This muscular valve between your esophagus and stomach is designed to shut tight after the food gets to the stomach to keep the stomach contents from sloshing backwards, or *refluxing,* into your esophagus.

The single test used to measure the strength of your esophageal muscles and/or the pressure exerted at the LES is called *esophageal manometry.* This test is rarely needed, unless antireflux surgery (see Chapter 12) is being considered or you have problems swallowing.

Preparing for this test

Don't consume food and liquids for 12 hours before the test. Don't take any antacids, antireflux medicines, alcohol, antidepressants, antihistamines, anti-Parkinson drugs, antispasmodics, muscle relaxants, and steroid drugs for 24 hours before the test.

Again, discuss continuing or stopping any medications with your doctor.

Taking this test

The doctor or medical technician running this test passes a thin tube in through your nose, down the back of your throat, and into your esophagus. With the tube in place, you take sips of water and swallow. As you do, electronic sensors on the tube in your esophagus register the pressure in your esophagus as the muscular walls contract and relax and the LES opens and closes. This information is transmitted to a recorder at the end of the tube protruding from your nose, which is removed, of course, after the test is over — the recorder and tube, not your nose!

Evaluating the results

A test showing reduced muscle power enables the surgeon to evaluate whether a patient will benefit from heartburn surgery, a procedure that narrows the esophagus, so that a patient's esophageal muscles can contract strongly enough to push food through the narrowed opening. See Chapter 12 for a complete description of surgeries.

Abnormal pressure at the LES suggests a malfunctioning valve, thus supporting a diagnosis of GERD.

Studying Your Stomach

The normal progression of the food you eat is from your mouth, to your esophagus, your stomach, your small intestine, your large intestine, your anus, and out. For some people, this process slows down, so that the stomach stays full longer. A full stomach pushes up against the LES, which may pop open at the wrong time, allowing acid stomach contents to flow backwards into the esophagus.

Gastric emptying studies show how quickly (or how slowly) the stomach empties after you eat. Doctors don't usually perform this test, except for GERD patients who also have other medical conditions (diabetes most commonly) that affect stomach emptying. In addition, if you have a lot of nausea or vomiting with your reflux, knowing how your stomach empties may be helpful to your doctor.

Preparing for this test

Don't consume food and liquids for 12 hours before the test. Your doctor may want to stop or change some of your medications prior to the test, so this is another time to discuss things with her ahead of time.

Taking this test

You eat a meal that contains a radioactive substance. The doctor or radiological technician running the test places a sensor, which reacts to radioactive material, over your stomach. The sensor takes pictures that tell if the radioactive material is in your stomach and when the food moves on, thus enabling the technician to figure out how long food lingers in your tummy. There are many different ways to do the test, which vary from hospital to hospital.

Evaluating the results

If your stomach empties more slowly than normal and your doctor is sure that you have acid reflux disease, he may prescribe medicines that speed up the process.

Evaluating Your Esophagus

When you're talking about tests, this section is the Big Time for your esophagus. To reach this level of testing, you must exhibit symptoms of GERD which suggest esophageal damage that requires your doctor take a closer look with one or more of the three following tests:

- ✔ A **barium swallow,** a noninvasive radiological examination of your esophageal lining

- ✔ An **upper GI (gastrointestinal) series,** a noninvasive radiological examination of your esophagus, stomach, and small intestine

- ✔ An **esophageal endoscopy,** an invasive examination of the esophagus that permits the doctor to take a tissue sample for a biopsy

These tests are listed in order of complexity. Which one (or more) your doctor orders is up to him.

Barium swallow

The barium swallow is most often done for people who have frequent reflux or difficulty swallowing. The test requires you to sip a solution of the metallic element barium in water. When you drink the liquid, the barium coats all the teensy little folds and crevices of your esophageal lining, making them visible to a *fluoroscope,* a device that shows a real-time image created by X-rays passing through the body.

Preparing for this test
Don't consume any food or liquids for at least 12 hours before the test.

Taking this test
To take this test, you

1. Stand behind a fluoroscopic screen.

2. Take swallows of a barium liquid.

3. Have pictures taken to show how the liquid moves from your mouth to your *pharynx* (the opening at the back of your mouth) and your esophagus, and how it flows down the esophagus.

Sometimes you may be asked to swallow a soft barium "marshmallow" (white bread soaked in barium liquid), which shows up as solid material passing through your gut. This is more often done when a patient has trouble with swallowing.

Talkin' the (radiology) talk

Medical specialists often have their very own language. For example, radiologists use the following terms to describe specific radiological tests:

X-ray: A picture created by exposing the body to ionizing radiation (radiation that can separate the atoms that make up any individual molecule)

Fluoroscope: A device that shows a real-time image created by X-rays passing through the body

Cineradiography: A technique that produces an X-ray moving picture of an organ or system such as the gastrointestinal tract at work

---

Evaluating the result

Pictures showing smooth, even distribution of the barium liquid over the lining of the pharynx and the esophagus say your esophagus is healthy.

Abnormalities in the distribution of the barium liquid may show the following GERD-related problems (for more on the symptoms and signs of GERD, check out Chapter 3):

- Esophageal muscle weakness, a known risk factor for GERD
- Esophageal *stricture*, narrowing of the esophagus due to repeated exposure to acid reflux
- Esophageal tumors, which may (or may not) be malignant
- Esophageal *ulcers*, reflux-related erosion of the surface of the esophagus
- Hiatal hernia (see Chapter 4)

Upper GI series

The upper GI series is a fluoroscopic examination of the esophagus, stomach, and small intestine. This test looks for the same kinds of problems as a barium swallow, but the upper GI — for **g**astro**i**ntestinal — series covers more intestinal acreage.

This test is usually recommended for people who have

- Difficulty moving food down the esophagus or pain while swallowing
- Frequent reflux and heartburn, plus such symptoms of stomach or small bowel disease such as nausea, vomiting, diarrhea, weight loss, or bleeding

Preparing for this test

Eat a low *residue* (dietary fiber) diet for two to three days before the test. Don't consume any food or liquids for 12 hours before the test.

Taking this test

You swallow a barium solution. Then you lie on a tilting table that is first positioned to enable a technician to do a fluoroscopic exam while you're in standing position.

Then the technician turns the table to different angles and positions in order to make different parts of your upper digestive system visible to the fluoroscopic camera.

Evaluating the results

A smooth distribution of the barium solution over the lining of the esophagus, stomach, and small intestine shows a healthy upper GI tract, meaning you may have GERD but don't have any visible reflux-related damage to your gastrointestinal tract.

Unusual or uneven distribution of the barium solution may show

- Esophageal muscle weakness

- Esophageal strictures

- Esophageal tumors, which may (or may not) be malignant

- Esophageal ulcers

- Hiatal hernia (for more, check out Chapter 4)

Upper endoscopy

If the barium swallow or the upper GI series shows abnormalities on the surface of the esophagus, your doctor may recommend an *upper endoscopy*. This test has the advantage of enabling the doctor to look directly at the esophageal tissue and to obtain tissue samples for biopsy so as to determine whether cells in the tissue are *malignant* (cancerous).

Your doctor may also recommend an upper endoscopy for people whose symptoms are the same as those in the section "Upper GI series," earlier in this chapter.

In fact, many guideline statements (including the official guideline statement of the American College of Gastroenterology, written by the contributing author of this very book) suggest that upper endoscopy is actually the first test to do if the patient is at risk for reflux complications. Its big advantage over radiology is that tissue samples (*biopsies*) can be performed with endoscopy.

Preparing for this test

Don't consume food or liquids for 12 hours prior to the test. Certain blood thinners may also need to be stopped prior to the test.

Taking this test

The person performing the endoscopy sprays your throat to numb it and then, as you can see in Figure 9-1, slides a thin, flexible plastic tube called an *endoscope* down your mouth into your esophagus.

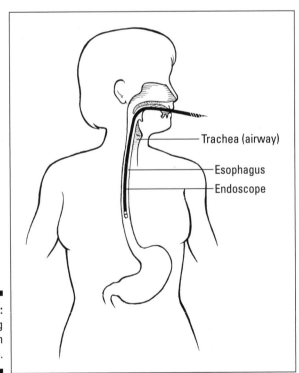

Trachea (airway)

Esophagus
Endoscope

Figure 9-1:
Scoping
out an
endoscope.

The endoscope has a tiny camera that transmits an image to a television screen where the doctor can visualize the esophageal lining. If he sees something unusual, such as a growth on the tissue, the doctor may also use small tweezerlike forceps in the endoscope to take a sample for a biopsy. No, you don't feel a thing — you don't have any nerve endings in your esophagus that say "ouch" when the doctor takes the sample.

If the endoscopy shows a narrowing of the esophagus, the doctor may insert a balloon or other stretching device through the endoscope and inflate it inside your esophagus to _dilate_ (stretch) the tube right on the spot. Afterwards, your esophagus will stay stretched, making it easier for you to swallow.

Evaluating the results

Smooth, undisturbed tissue shows a healthy esophageal lining. In other words, you may have GERD, but it hasn't damaged your esophagus.

A biopsy of esophageal tissue can diagnose conditions such as

- ✔ Bacterial or viral infection
- ✔ Damage cause by acid reflux
- ✔ Precancerous or malignant changes in esophageal cells

With diagnosis in hand, your doctor can begin to treat these problems.

Chapter 10

Prescribing Relief

· ·

In This Chapter

▶ Listing antireflux drugs

▶ Examining antacids

▶ Thwarting your reflux with blockers

▶ Stopping reflux at the pump

▶ Tracking interactions

· ·

*S*top! If you're reading this chapter before you read Chapter 6, you may want to skip back and read that one first because your initial attempt to control your heartburn/reflux should almost certainly involve dietary considerations. Why? Because there's always the delicious possibility that simply eliminating one specific food from your regular menu or changing your eating habits (hint: smaller meals) may squelch the burning sensation in your gullet.

If you've already gone the food route and your doctor says, "Time to pop some pills" — or, more likely, "Maybe we should try medication" — this chapter is a hands-on guide to over-the-counter (OTC) and prescription reflux remedies. Use it, and (hopefully) lose it — this chapter and your heartburn, respectively.

Noting the Cost of Heartburn Help

Every year, Americans cough up more than $1 billion for OTC heartburn remedies and as much as $6 billion (yes, billion!) for just one prescription product, omeprazole (Prilosec). Kinda stops you in your tracks to think that Americans spend more on meds to relieve a pain in the gut than several dozen nations may spend on their whole darn gross national product.

Of course, reflux isn't just a simple pain in the middle. Treating the symptoms effectively can reduce the risk of potentially fatal complications, such as cancer, later on (see Chapter 3).

Drugs versus medicines

What's the difference between *a drug* and *a medicine?* Scientifically speaking, nothing. In fact, *Webster's New World College Dictionary* (Wiley) defines *medicine* as *any drug.*

Grammatically, however, the difference is pronounced. The word *drug* may serve either as a noun or a verb (as in "to drug someone"), but the verb for *medicine* is *to medicate.* And talk about your culture wars: Unless you've missed every shoot-'em-up, chase-'em-down, cops 'n' robbers TV show or movie of the past half century, you know the word *drug* can have unpleasant connotations that *medicine* doesn't have — like, oh, *drug dealer, drug trade,* or *druggie.*

In other words, when you're talking drugs, if you mean medicine, sometimes it helps to say so. Unless, that is, you're writing Chapter 10 in *Heartburn & Reflux For Dummies* in which I use *drug* once in a while in place of a *medicine,* or even *meds,* for a little variety.

Making the decision to buy and use meds that can make your reflux-related heartburn less painful and less damaging to your esophagus — and maybe even eliminate heartburn and reflux entirely — is a sensible choice.

The medicines I examine in this chapter can be neatly classified as belonging to one of three broad categories:

- Antacids
- Histamine 2 receptor blockers, also known as *H2 blockers*
- Proton pump inhibitors (PPIs)

As you may expect, each group has its very own special benefits and annoyances, so I want to run down the list, one category at a time, to figure out which may be the best choice for you.

After you have this info, you'll confirm the choice with your doctor, right? Of course, you will. Forgive me for even asking. But I give you fair warning that the words "check with your doctor" appear many times in this chapter. When you're coping with a potentially serious condition such as heartburn/reflux — and whenever the subject turns to medications — your doctor is an invaluable guide through an often confusing medical maze.

Aiming for Neutrality with Antacids

On any given day, after any given meal, your stomach pumps out acid like there's no tomorrow in order to break down, digest, and grab nutrients out of the various kinds of food you so casually toss down there. As a result, your stomach's contents are very acidic. Not too acidic for your stomach, mind you, because your stomach lining is tough enough to resist the burn.

But if the stomach gunk accidentally refluxes (splashes back) through your lower esophageal sphincter (LES) — the muscular ring that is supposed to shut tight after you swallow to keep stomach contents safely in your stomach — you'll know right away. Why? Because your esophageal lining is more delicate than your stomach lining. When acid hits your esophageal lining, it hurts.

OTC antacids are your first line of defense.

Describing how antacids help

Antacids are *bases,* the chemical opposite of *acids.* Basic compounds, such as antacids, neutralize acidic solutions, such as the reflux in your esophagus.

pH is a scale used to measure the acidity of solutions, such as stomach acid, coffee, or drain cleaner. Acids are at the low end of the numbers on the pH scale; bases at the high end. You can read all about pH, acids, and bases in Chapter 2. For now, all you need to do is memorize this simple formula:

Acid + Base = Neutral = Pain relief

Antacids neutralize reflux that sloshes back through the LES and into your esophagus, but they (the antacids) don't inhibit your stomach's natural and necessary secretion of acids. So, antacids don't stop your stomach from secreting acids to digest food, nor do they totally neutralize the acidity of stomach contents. But they can do a pretty good job of making your stomach contents less irritating to your esophagus. The gastro gurus who have taken the time to measure this reaction say antacids may neutralize up to 99 percent of the acids in the reflux in your esophagus.

Ah, but antacids have a few more tricks up their sleeves when it comes to fighting heartburn:

✔ Antacids also slow down the activation of *pepsin,* one of your stomach's natural digestive enzymes. Cutting the activity of pepsin is important because like the Roman god Janus, pepsin has two faces — one good, one not so good.

 • In your stomach, pepsin helps digest food proteins (yeah!).

 • In your esophagus, pepsin may damage the surface of the esophageal lining (boo!).

✔ Antacids may stimulate the stomach's natural production of

- **Bicarbonates:** Natural antacids, which neutralize stomach acids.

- **Mucus:** A substance that protects the lining of the stomach.

- **Prostaglandins:** Naturally occurring compounds that influence the expansion and contraction of *smooth muscle,* the type of muscle found in the lining of your blood vessels, organs such as the uterus and your intestines, and, of course, your LES.

And that is why the authors of the American Pharmaceutical Association's *Handbook of Nonprescription Drugs* believe that antacids may also strengthen the muscle tone of the LES, helping to keep it closed and reducing the risk of reflux.

The opposite of smooth muscle is *striated muscle,* the kind of tissue found in your skeletal muscles, such as your biceps, your triceps, your abs, and so on. Did you take Biology or Physiology 101? You may have seen the difference through a microscope, which shows smooth muscle tissue as smooth (surprise!) and striated muscle with that look like lines (*striations*) running across it.

Naming the antacid ingredients in antacid products

Read the labels carefully, and you can see that the ingredients in antacids have common mineral names. Why? Because minerals such as the following are — yes, you guessed it — bases.

Side versus adverse: The effective difference

Side effects are normal, totally expected consequences of taking a medicine. For example, if you take the antidepressant paroxetine (Paxil), some people may *normally expect* to feel drowsy.

Adverse effects, on the other hand, are unexpected, unusual, infrequent, and possibly serious reactions. For example, when you pop that paroxetine, you don't *normally expect* to develop an allergic rash or respiratory problem.

Considering how depressingly adverse it would be to develop a rash or have breathing difficulty after taking an antidepressant, you can see from this example that a side effect is generally annoying but nonthreatening, while an adverse effect may require immediate medical attention — or at least a phone call to your doctor.

Sodium bicarbonate

Sodium bicarbonate, better known as *baking soda* to bakers and nonbakers alike, is a star ingredient in antacid products. The white powder dissolves quick as a wink in water. As soon as you swallow, a bicarbonate solution immediately neutralizes acid in a reaction whose most prominent result is the release of carbon dioxide, a gas that makes you burp.

Drawback: Sodium bicarbonate is high in sodium, which means that people on low-sodium diets may be directed to avoid products containing it. Chapter 7 describes sodium bicarbonate as a home remedy.

Calcium carbonate

Calcium carbonate is a potent acid neutralizer with an extra benefit: calcium, as in bone-building, osteoporosis-fighting calcium.

Drawback: Calcium carbonate may be constipating.

Aluminum compounds

Aluminum compounds, such as aluminum hydroxide, are also effective acid neutralizers.

Drawbacks: Aluminum compounds are slow to dissolve and slow to start working. In addition, large amounts of aluminum compounds hook up to phosphates (phosphorus compounds) in various parts of your body, including your bones. As a result, people who are malnourished may begin to lose phosphorous from their bones. Finally, aluminum compounds may not be safe for people with kidney disease. And did I mention that the most frequent side effect of aluminum compounds is constipation? Forewarned is forearmed, as they say.

Magnesium compounds

Magnesium compounds, such as magnesium hydroxide and magnesium trisilicate, are safe and effective acid neutralizers for healthy people.

Drawbacks: Magnesium compounds aren't recommended for people with kidney disease. In addition, they may cause diarrhea.

Aluminum/magnesium combinations

Aluminum/magnesium combinations are also effective acid neutralizers.

Drawbacks: These combinations also offer up the side effects of both products: Possible constipation from the aluminum and diarrhea from the magnesium. Theoretically, this should strike a happy balance, but whom am I kidding? Medical experience suggests that diarrhea predominates, especially if you exceed the recommended dose of a combination product.

Citric acid and tartaric aid

A compound with the word *acid* in its name hardly seems like an antacid, but both citric acid and tartaric acid do act as antacids, and, for good measure, both are flavoring agents.

Drawback: Some individuals may be sensitive to citric acid. One possible reaction: Chapped or peeling lips.

Reviewing other ingredients in antacid products

Architect Ludwig Mies van der Rohe, the designer of the glorious bronze Seagram Building on Park Avenue in New York City, summed up his philosophy in three little words. No, no, not "I love you." Mies' wonderfully wise words were: "Less is more."

Unfortunately, modern med marketers seem to have missed Mies' point. On the drugstore shelf, less is always less, while more is definitely more. As in "more complicated," "more possibility of side effects," and don't forget, "more expensive." Following is a list of some of the "more" ingredients you may find in your antacid.

- ✔ **Analgesics:** Aspirin and acetaminophen are sometimes included to relieve a headache linked to an upset stomach.

  Drawback: Aspirin upsets some sensitive tummies. Acetaminophen doesn't.

- ✔ **Foaming agent:** *Alginic acid* (sodium alginate) puffs up into a foamy barrier around your LES. This barrier is most helpful for people with a *hiatal hernia,* your stomach's bulging through a gap in the muscle around the LES (read more about hiatal hernias in Chapter 4).

  Drawback: An alginic acid foam floats on top of the liquids in your stomach so — now picture this clearly in your mind's eye — you have to be upright for the foam to create a barrier around the LES. In other words, don't take an antacid product containing alginic acid when you lie down.

- ✔ **Gas guzzler:** Simethicone is an *antiflatulant,* an ingredient that breaks up intestinal gas. Some studies show that it works; others show no effect. No bloating with your reflux? Skip the simethicone.

  Drawbacks: None. Isn't that nice?

✔ **Sodium:** Most antacids contain some sodium but some antacids contain lots of sodium.

Drawback: If you're on a low-sodium diet, read antacid labels *very* carefully. Or, heck, just take the easy way: Ask your doctor if the product belongs in your personal medicine chest.

Can't keep track of the players without a scorecard? Check out Table 10-1 for the basic stats of some commonly available OTC products that contain one or more of the ingredients I've just described. For your convenience, I've included toll-free numbers and Web sites (where available) for more info.

Table 10-1	Examining Antacids			
Brand-Name (Dose)	Antacid Ingredient(s)	Other Active Ingredient(s)	Toll-Free Number	Web Site
Alka-Seltzer				
Tablet	Sodium bicarbonate (1,916 mg) Citric acid (1,000 mg)	Aspirin (325 mg)	800-800-4793	www.alka-seltzer.com
Brioschi				
1 capful	Sodium bicarbonate (2,690 mg) Tartaric acid (2,430 mg)		800-BRIOSCHI	www.brioschi-usa.com
Bromo Seltzer				
¾ capful	Sodium bicarbonate (2,781 mg) Citric acid (2,224 mg)	Acetaminophen (325 mg)		
Packet	Sodium bicarbonate (3,590 mg) Citric acid (2,679 mg)	Acetaminophen (650 mg)		

(continued)

Table 10-1 *(continued)*

Brand-Name (Dose)	Antacid Ingredient(s)	Other Active Ingredient(s)	Toll-Free Number	Web Site
Gaviscon Extra Strength				
Tablet	Aluminum hydroxide (160 mg) Magnesium carbonate (105 mg)	Alginic acid (listed as inactive ingredient; no amount given)	888-452-0051	www.gaviscon.com
Tsp/liquid	Aluminum hydroxide (254 mg) Magnesium carbonate (237.5 mg)	Alginic acid (listed as inactive ingredient; no amount given)	888-452-0051	www.gaviscon.com
Maalox Max				
Tsp/liquid	Aluminum hydroxide (409 mg) Magnesium hydroxide (400 mg)	Simethicone (40 mg)	800-452-0051	www.maaloxus.com
Tablet	Calcium carbonate (1,000 mg)	Simethicone (60 mg)	800-452-0051	www.maaloxus.com
Mylanta				
Tsp/liquid	Aluminum hydroxide (200 mg) Magnesium hydroxide (200 mg)	Simethicone (20 mg)	800-469-5268	www.mylanta.com
Rolaids Original				
Tablet	Calcium carbonate (550 mg) Magnesium hydroxide (110 mg)		800-223-0182	www.rolaids.com

Brand-Name (Dose)	Antacid Ingredient(s)	Other Active Ingredient(s)	Toll-Free Number	Web Site
Rolaids Multi-symptom				
Tablet	Calcium carbonate (675 mg) Magnesium hydroxide (135 mg)	Simethicone (60 mg)	800-223-0182	www.rolaids.com
Tums				
Tablet	Calcium carbonate (500 mg)			www.tums.com

Sources: Product labels, October 2003; Web sites.

Blocking the Burn

Okay. So you tried antacids and . . . nothing. Your heartburn's still smoldering more than two times a week, which means you qualify as a person with "frequent heartburn," which means your doctor may suggest a step up the antireflux drug ladder to *histamine 2 receptor antagonists,* better known as *H2 blockers.*

H2 blockers are compounds whose molecules glom onto *H2 receptors,* specific sites on the cells in the walls of your intestinal tract. This meeting of molecules and cells slows your stomach's secretion of acids, which makes your stomach contents less irritating when they splash back into your esophagus. No, H2 blockers don't prevent reflux; they simply reduce the amount of acid in your stomach.

And studies show that H2 blockers (like the protein pump inhibitors you can read about in "Slowing the Pump," later in this chapter) may have the ability to heal reflux-related damage to the lining of your esophagus. If further studies prove this to be true and show that the healing action is strong and reliable, taking these medicines may reduce the risk of reflux-related esophageal cancer. Stay tuned for the latest developments. Or just check with your doctor.

Right now, there are four — count 'em, four — H2 blockers on the market:

- Cimetidine (Tagamet), pronounced sy-*met*-ah-deen
- Famotidine (Pepcid), pronounced fah-*mo*-tah-deen
- Nizatidine (Axid), pronounced nih-*zah*-tah-deen
- Ranitidine (Zantac), pronounced rah-*nih*-tah-deen

Separating prescription and OTC H2 blockers

Each of the Fab Four is available as a prescription drug and as an OTC product. So what exactly are the differences between the two versions? Easy as pie: Usage, dosage, timing, problems, and — the 800-pound gorilla in the drugstore — cost.

- **Use:** Prescription H2 blockers are approved for treating gastrointestinal reflux disease (GERD) and other serious illnesses such as recurring peptic ulcers. The OTC products are meant for people who have heartburn only once in a while — a technical term that means less than twice a week.

- **Dosage:** Prescription-strength H2 blockers deliver up to four times as much medicine. For example, OTC cimetidine has 200 mg per tablet. Prescription cimetidine is available in 100 mg, 200 mg, 300 mg, 400 mg, 600 mg, and 800 mg.

- **Timing:** You take the OTC products as needed, like right before you're about to eat a humongous sausage hero sandwich washed down with beer. Or right after when your heartburn says, "Cure me! Now!" You take the prescription product on a regular schedule as a *maintenance drug,* a medicine used to treat a continuing condition.

- **Side effects and adverse effects:** The higher the dose, the more likely you are to have the problems spelled out in the following section on "Counting drawbacks." No surprise there.

- **Cost:** Prescription products cost more. No surprise there — unless you have a drug plan that pays for prescription meds but not those sold OTC, a problem you can read more about in "The OTC dilemma," a sidebar in this chapter.

Table 10-2 offers a quick comparison of OTC versus prescription-strength H2 blockers. Note that there are differences in some of the descriptions of how to use different H2 blockers. This may or may not be important. Many physicians and gastro researchers believe that so long as you're comparing prescription products with prescription products or OTC products with OTC products "an H2 blocker is an H2 blocker is an H2 blocker" and that you can use them interchangeably.

Pharmacies and drugstores sell H2 blockers without a prescription, but that doesn't mean these products aren't serious medicines. The OTC version is meant for simple heartburn; if you have reflux, you may need a prescription. So before setting your own dosing schedule, check with your doctor.

Table 10-2	Comparing H2 Blockers			
	Cimetidine	*Famotidine*	*Nizatidine*	*Ranitidine*
OTC Products (for Heartburn)				
Brand	Tagamet HB 200	Pepcid AC*	Axid AR	Zantac 75
Dosage (tablets)	200 mg	10 mg	75 mg	75 mg
How long it works	2.5 hours	4 hours	2 hours	3 hours
When to take this pill	30 minutes before eating	Before eating or when heartburn occurs	Twice a day	Twice a day unless specifically directed by your doctor
Prescription Products (for Reflux/GERD)				
Brand (U.S.)	Tagamet	Pepcid	Axid	Zantac
Brand (Canada)	Enlon, Peptol	Acid Control	Apo-Nizatidine	Zantac-C
Dosage (tablets)	100 mg, 200 mg, 300 mg, 400 mg, 600 mg, 800 mg	20 mg, 40 mg	75 mg, 150 mg, 300 mg**	150 mg
When to take this pill	4 × with meals or 1 × at bedtime	At bedtime	2 × daily	

Pepcid Complete (OTC) has famotidine plus two antacids, calcium carbonate (800mg/tablet) and magnesium hydroxide (165mg/tablet).
**Capsules*
Sources: Handbook of Nonprescription Drugs, *13th ed. (Washington D.C.: American Pharmaceutical Association, 2002);* James J. Rybacki, The Essential Guide to Prescription Drugs 2003 *(New York: Harper Collins, 2003).*

Counting drawbacks

Did you really think you were going to get out of this section without a few warnings? Of course not. Anyone savvy enough to buy *Heartburn & Reflux For Dummies* knows deep in his or her smart little heart that H2 blockers are likely to have a few annoying characteristics, such as how long they take to work, what they can't do even when they're working at top speed, and their unpleasant side effects and adverse effects.

So should everybody with heartburn take an H2 blocker? Not so fast. H2 blockers are more medicine than you need if you only have occasional heartburn. On the other hand, they may not be as effective as protein pump inhibitors (PPIs) if you have frequent reflux or GERD. This choice is for your doctor to make.

Timing your relief

H2 blockers take longer to swing into action than plain antacids do, but after they get going, the H2 blockers work stronger and longer, up to four hours for the H2 blockers compared to 30 minutes to an hour for the antacids. Hey, you lose some, you win some.

Posting the missing powers

H2 blockers don't make your LES stronger and unlike proton pump inhibitors, which I discuss later in this chapter, they don't cut back on the number of times you may experience reflux. In other words, you don't stop having reflux, but you do hurt less. I say it again: You win some, you lose some.

Adding up unpleasantries

H2 blockers have their own set of problems. The most likely side effects are pretty much what you may expect with tummy meds:

- Constipation or diarrhea
- Headache
- Nausea and vomiting
- Pain in the belly

The adverse effects of H2 blockers, which are definitely more adverse than the side effects, may include the following:

- Confusion, dizziness, and hallucinations
- Mild anemia
- Mild drop in blood pressure
- Slow heartbeat

Lucky for you, these pill problems are fairly uncommon. Overall, the incidence of side effects and adverse effects with H2 blockers is about 3 percent. Translation: About 3 of every 100 people who take an OTC or prescription H2 blocker experiences drug-related trouble. Did I mention you win some, you lose some?

Watching out for sex and reproduction

Scientists have linked some annoying, unpleasant, or downright hazardous interference with sexual prowess and reproductive functions to H2 blockers. Table 10-3 shows what I'm talking about.

This table contains some information regarding the safety of drugs for pregnant women and their developing fetuses. In 1979, the Food and Drug Administration (FDA) created five Pregnancy Risk Categories for drugs based on evidence from human pregnancy studies or studies of animal reproduction. The categories range from the safest (Category A) to the most hazardous (Category X). The FDA has assigned a rating to virtually every drug sold in the United States; health agencies in other countries have adopted similar ratings. The ratings in this chart are those assigned by the FDA to these drugs as of 2003.

Table 10-3	Sex and the Single H2 Blocker
Drug (Population)	**Comments**
Cimetidine	
Men and women	Long-term use may cause breast swelling and tenderness.
Men	May be linked to male impotence (rare).
	May be linked to lower sperm counts.
Women	Rated Category B for pregnant women, which means either that studies show no evidence of damage to animal fetuses but no well-controlled studies in human beings *or* that animal reproductive studies show fetal abnormalities but well-controlled studies show no risk to the human fetus.
	Although H2 blockers pass into breast milk, the American Academy of Pediatrics rated cimetidine Category B for pregnant women, which means either that studies show no evidence of damage to animal fetuses but no well-controlled studies in human beings *or* that animal reproductive studies show fetal abnormalities but doesn't consider this med a risk to the infant.

(continued)

Table 10-3 *(continued)*

Drug (Population)	Comments
Famotidine	
Men	May be linked to male impotence (rare).
Women	Well-controlled studies show no risk to the human fetus.
	Although H2 blockers pass into breast milk, the American Academy of Pediatrics doesn't consider this med a risk to the infant.
Nizatidine	
Men and women	Long-term use may cause breast swelling and tenderness.
Men	May be linked to male impotence (rare).
Women	Has been associated with a higher incidence of spontaneous abortion in laboratory rabbits and is rated Category C for pregnant women, which means that reproductive studies show damage to both animal and human fetuses *or* that the dangers to the fetus outweigh the possible benefits of the drug.
	Although H2 blockers pass into breast milk, the American Academy of Pediatrics doesn't consider this med a risk to the infant.
Ranitidine	
Men and women	Long-term use may cause breast swelling and tenderness.
Women	Rated Category B for Category B for pregnant women, which means either that studies show no evidence of damage to animal fetuses but no well-controlled studies in human beings *or* that animal reproductive studies show fetal abnormalities but well-controlled studies show no risk to the human fetus.
	Although H2 blockers pass into breast milk, the American Academy of Pediatrics doesn't consider this med a risk to the infant.

Sources: Handbook of Nonprescription Drugs, *13th ed. (Washington D.C.: American Pharmaceutical Association, 2002); James J. Rybacki,* The Essential Guide to Prescription Drugs 2003 *(New York: Harper Collins, 2003).*

Help! My reflux medicine is giving me allergies!

In the fall of 2003, the British Broadcasting Corporation announced that researchers at the University of Vienna had stumbled across an unexpected adverse effect among volunteers taking the H2 blocker ranitidine: Allergies. Not to the H2 blocker, mind you, but to foods.

In a study with about 300 volunteers, food allergies were more common among the folks taking ranitidine than among those taking a look-alike placebo pill. The professors proposed that ranitidine's ability to slow the production of stomach acid may have interrupted the natural digestion of food, allowing allergens to slide pretty much whole from the stomach to small intestine, thus provoking the aforementioned allergies.

Slowing the Pump

Proton pump inhibitors, also known as PPIs, are the new Wow! in the war on reflux. Right now, your doctor can pull any one of five PPIs out of his pharmacopoeia (pronounced far-mah-co-*pee*-ah) — a medically musical way of saying *list of available drugs.* The five are

- ✔ Omeprazole (Prilosec/introduced in 1986)
- ✔ Lansoprazole (Prevacid/introduced in 1995)
- ✔ Rabeprazole (Aciphex/introduced in 1999)
- ✔ Pantoprazole (Protonix/introduced in 2001)
- ✔ Esomeprazole (Nexium/introduced in 2001)

Several studies suggest that in addition to effectively reducing the production of stomach acid, PPIs may also help heal reflux-related esophageal injuries. If you're scratching your head and muttering, "Hey, that sounds a lot like H2 blockers" — which I described in the previous section — guess what? You're right. If future studies confirm that PPIs are healers as well as acid-reducers, that would be big news.

But that doesn't mean that H2 blockers and PPIs are exactly alike. They aren't. The differences? PPIs are

- ✔ More effective than H2 blockers at reducing acid production and keeping the level low for relatively long periods of time
- ✔ More effective than H2 blockers at healing reflux-damaged esophageal tissue

Defining PPIs

So what's a PPI anyway? Sometimes the name says it all, although you may need a medical dictionary to translate what the words mean. Like:

Proton pump inhibitors are compounds that

> *Inhibit* the activity of an enzyme — (H+, K+)-ATPase, to be exact — containing
>
> *Protons* (positively charged particles) that enables special cells in your stomach wall to
>
> *Pump* out stomach acids

I can't leave this paragraph without telling you that H=hydrogen, K=potassium, ATP=adenosine 5-triphosphate, and *-ase* is the suffix that means *enzyme.* Aren't you glad you know that?

PPIs don't neutralize stomach acid (as antacids do) or simply slow its production (as H2 blockers do). They actually wipe out some of that pesky stomach enzyme, reducing the amount of acid your stomach can make for as long as it takes your body to build more of the enabling enzyme. Depending on which PPI your doctor prescribes, you can expect your pill to

✔ Begin wiping out enzymes 2 to 5 minutes after you take it

✔ Hit its highest levels in your blood in anywhere from 30 minutes to an hour or two

✔ Give you relief that may last all day

These benefits sure beat both antacids and H2 blockers. Do I hear you saying, "Tell me more?" My pleasure.

Comparing PPIs

As you can see, the names of all PPIs end in *–prazole* (pronounced *prah*-zoll), signifying that they're pharmaceutical cousins. But even close relatives may have differences, so you'd expect that doctors would know which PPI

✔ Goes to work fastest

✔ Gives the longest pain relief

✔ Heals injured tissues most effectively

Table 10-4 does give you an overview of these medicines, but, beware! With the exception of omeprazole, which has been around since 1986, PPIs are relatively new. Although researchers have conducted some head-to-head comparison studies, the evidence can be conflicting.

For example, in October 2003, *U.S. Pharmacist,* a trade magazine for (who else?) pharmacists, noted that

- ✔ Some clinical trials show that 30 mg lansoprazole works faster than 20 mg omeprazole.

- ✔ Some clinical trials show that 40 mg esomeprazole provides relief faster and heals esophageal tissue damage more completely than 20 mg omeprazole.

- ✔ Some studies suggest that 20 mg rabeprazole keeps stomach acidity lower twice as long as 20 mg omeprazole.

- ✔ Esomeprazole 40 mg chased reflux symptoms better than 30 mg lansoprazole.

- ✔ Other studies show no differences — that's right, no differences — among the drugs.

- ✔ Some studies that show differences depict them as so small (like 4 percent) that they aren't considered significant.

As a result, much of what you may hear right now about PPIs is anecdotal, as in "My sister-in-law's brother had been using PPI (A), and then his doctor gave him a prescription for PPI (B) and he, the brother that is, says PPI (B) worked much faster for him." Or slower.

Sooner or later more hard facts will be available rather than stories about friends and relatives to show exactly how good the various PPIs are. For now, your best source on updates and news about PPIs is your doctor. Table 10-4 gives you some benchmarks on prescription PPI pill behavior, but remember that what you read in this table is hardly the last word.

Omeprazole (Prilosec) is available as an OTC medicine called (surprise!) Prilosec OTC. Prescription Prilosec comes in several dosages; but both prescription omeprazole and OTC omeprazole come in 20-mg tablets, so the information in Table 10-4 compares effects for the 20-mg size of both.

Table 10-4	Comparing PPI Pill Products		
PPI	*Brand Name*	*Dose**	*Hits Highest Blood Levels In*
Omeprazole**	Prilosec	20 mg	0.5–3.5 hours
Lansoprazole	Prevacid	30 mg	1.7 hours

(continued)

Table 10-4 *(continued)*

PPI	Brand Name	Dose*	Hits Highest Blood Levels In
Rabeprazole	Aciphex	20 mg	2–5 hours
Pantoprazole	Protonix	40 mg	1–3 hours
Esomeprazole	Nexium	40 mg	1.6 hours

*The customary dose for reflux is one pill, once a day.
**Available both as a prescription drug and as an OTC product.
Sources: *Margarita V. DiVall, "The Role of Proton Pump Inhibitors in the Management of GERD,"* U.S. Pharmacist, *October 2003; Sarah Johnson, "UIHC: Proton Pump Inhibitors...An Update" (*www.vh.org/adult/provider/pharmacyservices/Gastrogram/2001Spring.html*); James J. Rybacki,* The Essential Guide to Prescription Drugs 2003 *(New York: Harper Collins, 2003).*

Listing potential problems

What a downer! After telling you how useful PPIs are, now I have to tack on some warnings about side effects and adverse effects.

Listing the side effects is like following Claude Rains's order in *Casablanca* to "round up the usual suspects." In this case, the most common side effects are

- Headache
- Diarrhea
- Indigestion
- Stomachache

All these side effects made at least a momentary appearance among volunteers in the October 2003 *U.S. Pharmaceutical* article.

The list of adverse effects includes the following:

- Anemias
- Chest or face pain
- Liver damage
- Low blood sugar
- Male breast enlargement
- Rare reports of allergic rashes and itching
- Yeast infections

The OTC dilemma

To OTC or not to OTC. That is the question. As world travelers know, many valuable drugs sold only on prescription in the United States are prescription-free abroad. Some people think that if the British, French, and Germans can handle serious meds, Americans can, too. Others say everyone in every country needs a physician to make an accurate diagnosis and to provide accurate information about how to avoid mistakes such as failing to match the right drug to the disease or failing to stay the therapeutic course, a potentially devastating decision. For example, if you stop taking an antibiotic too soon because you feel better, you may have wounded but not killed an infectious organism that adapts to fight another day, like when you try the same antibiotic a second time.

In the spring of 2003 when omeprazole morphed from prescription Prilosec to OTC Prilosec, the new OTC package attempted to forestall treatment problems by printing label copy with specific instructions to try just one 14-day course and call the doctor if the pills didn't relieve heartburn.

But will patients who don't get perfect relief make the call? Will they simply try another 14-day course, risking damage from continuing reflux? Will doctors find out before a serious problem surfaces? The answers, respectively, are: Who knows? Who knows? And, oh, yes, who knows?

The second bump on the prescription-to-OTC road is financial. OTC products aren't necessarily a cents-ible solution. As a prescription drug, omeprazole has been covered by many insurance plans. As an OTC product, it isn't. Folks who had been handing over a $5 or $10 copay soon found they had to pony up three times as much for a one-month supply. You're probably thinking that competition will lower the price. That remains to be seen, but, in some parts of the country, insurance companies are beginning to limit their payment for prescription PPIs and asking their patients to take the OTC (sometimes the insurance pays part of the cost; other times not). How this all sorts itself out is anybody's guess.

Right now, the Consumer Healthcare Products Association (CHPA) pooh-poohs concern about costs. Contrary to what its name implies, the CHPA isn't a consumer group but an alliance of companies that make OTC drugs. And you say, that explains the CHPA's statement that because most prescription drugs cost more than $40 a refill, while most OTC products cost less than $20 and because so many Americans don't have health insurance, the switch is a net plus for buyers.

In fact, between 1976 and 2003 the Food and Drug Administration (FDA) approved the prescription-to-OTC switch for 89 drug ingredients, combinations, and dosages (approving one ingredient in 10-mg and 20-mg sizes counts as two switches; who would figure?) resulting in more than 700 new products, such as antihistamines, fungus busters, hair restorers, painkillers, and, of course, antireflux meds that you can simply waltz into your drugstore and pluck off the shelf.

The truly curious may want to check out the whole list of switched drugs on the CPHA Web site at www.chpa-info.org. Or consider investing in an accessible reference book such as *The Essential Guide to Prescription Drugs* so often mentioned in this book.

However, the PPIs are mostly so new that these reports by people using the PPIs may not have been confirmed by well-controlled scientific studies. In other words, nobody knows for certain just which adverse effects are really more common than others.

Pregnant and nursing mothers have a few more things to look out for.

✔ Omeprazole has caused fetal deaths in laboratory rats and rabbits, so it's rated Category C for pregnant women, meaning that animal reproductive studies have shown fetal abnormalities but there are no well-controlled studies for human beings *or* there is no information from studies on either animals or human beings so that risk to the fetus can't be ruled out.

✔ The other four PPIs are ranked Category B for pregnant women, which means either that studies show no evidence of damage to animal fetuses but no well-controlled studies in human beings *or* that animal reproductive studies show fetal abnormalities but well-controlled studies show no risk to the human fetus

✔ All PPIs pass into breast milk, so these drugs aren't recommended for nursing mothers *without a doctor's advice.*

Interesting Interacting

What a pickle! One medical problem nicely under control thanks to your doctor's prescribing a perfectly peachy med, when another condition makes its way onto center stage: The dreaded interaction.

As Table 10-5 makes perfectly clear, antiheartburn/reflux products are no exception. Do I need to write again that you should always check with your doctor before starting to use an antacid, an H2 blocker, or a PPI?

Look carefully at Table 10-5 and you can see that I list several interactions for cimetidine and none at all for the other three H2 blockers. Why? Because cimetidine's chemical structure enables it to lock onto and inactivate several enzymes your body needs to metabolize various other drugs. Famotidine, nizatidine, and ranitidine don't behave this way.

Look again. You may notice many more interactions for omeprazole than for the other four PPIs. For the moment, just accept the fact that although the PPIs have similar chemical structures, omeprazole seems more likely to interact with other drugs. On the other hand, all the current studies show the five PPIs are similar in safety and effectiveness, which means that good old omeprazole may get blamed for more side effects just because it has been around longer.

In the end, let your doctor be your guide.

Table 10-5 is only a representative listing of the interactions that may occur between commonly used medicines and antiheartburn/reflux drugs. Information about drug side effects, adverse effects, and interactions is always a work in progress. As doctors discover more about new drugs, including new drugs for heartburn, additional information about interactions may surface. Who knows what nastiness will turn up tomorrow? Not me. Not you. And worst of all, not necessarily the folks who make, market, and prescribe medicines. As a result, this chart is a work in progress, a guide to current knowledge about interactions between heartburn medicines and other drugs. Check with your doctor for the most up-to-date info.

Table 10-5	Interacting: Heartburn/Reflux Meds and Other Drugs	
This Heartburn/ Reflux Drug	**Interacts with: Generic Name (Brand Name)**	**Used to Treat This Condition**
Antacids		
Aluminum compounds	Allopurinol (1)	Gout
	Atenolol (1)	Heart disease
	Cimetidine (Tagamet)	Heartburn/reflux
	Diazapam (Valium)	Anxiety
	Digoxin (Lanoxin)	Heart disease
	Isoniazid (INH)	Tuberculosis
	Ketoconazole (Nizoral)	Fungal infection
	Metoprolol (Lopressor)	Heart disease
	Prednisone (1)	Inflammation
	Propranolol (Inderal)	Heart disease
	Ranitidine (Zantac)	Reflux
	Sucralfate (Carafate)	Gastric ulcer
	Tetracyclines (1)	Bacterial infection
	Valproic acid (Depakene)	Seizures

(continued)

Table 10-5 *(continued)*

This Heartburn/ Reflux Drug	Interacts with: Generic Name (Brand Name)	Used to Treat This Condition
Calcium compounds	Ketoconazole (Nizoral)	Fungal infection
	Quinidine (Duroquin)	Irregular heartbeat
	Sucralfate (Carafate)	Gastric ulcer
	Tetracyclines (1)	Infections
Magnesium compounds	Digoxin (Lanoxin)	Heart disease
	Isoniazid (INF)	Tuberculosis
	Phenytoin (Dilantin)	Seizures
	Sucralfate (Carafate)	Gastric ulcer
	Tetracyclines (1)	Bacterial infection
	Valproic acid (Depakene)	Seizures
	Warfarin (Coumadin)	Blood-clotting problems
Aluminum/Magnesium combinations	Allopurinol (1)	Gout
	Atenalol (1)	Heart disease
	Cimetidine (Tagamet)	Heartburn/reflux
	Digoxin (Lanoxin)	Heart disease
	Ketoconazole (Nizoral)	Fungal infection
	Metoprolol (Lopressor)	Heart disease
	Prednisone (1)	Inflammation
	Ranitidine (Zantac)	Heartburn/reflux
	Sucralfate (Carafate)	Gastric ulcer
	Tetracyclines (1)	Bacterial infection
	Valproic acid (Depakene)	Seizures
Sodium bicarbonate	Ketoconazole (Nizoral)	Fungal infection
	Quinidine (Duroquin)	Irregular heartbeat
	Sucralfate (Carafate)	Gastric ulcer

This Heartburn/ Reflux Drug	Interacts with: Generic Name (Brand Name)	Used to Treat This Condition
H2 Blockers		
Cimetidine	Amitriptyline (Elavil) (2)	Depression
	Calcium channel blockers (3)	Heart disease
	Ketoconazole (Nizoral)	Fungal infections
	Phenytoin (Dilantin)	Seizures
	Quinidine (Duroquin)	Irregular heartbeat
	Theophylline (1)	Asthma
	Warfarin (Coumadin)	Blood-clotting problems
Famotidine	No significant interactions	
Nizatidine	No significant interactions	
Ranitidine	No significant interactions	
Proton Pump Inhibitors		
Esomeprazole	Diazepam (Valium)	Anxiety
	Ketoconazole (Nizoral)	Fungal infection
Lansoprazole	Ketoconazole (Nizoral)	Fungal infection
	Theophylline (1)	Asthma
Omeprazole	Carbamazepine (Tegretol)	Seizures
	Diazapam (Valium)	Anxiety
	Digoxin (Lanoxin)	Heart disease
	Ketoconazole (Nizoral)	Fungal infection
	Methotrexate (Mexate)	Psoriasis
	Nifedipine (Procardia)	Hypertension
	Phenytoin (Dilantin)	Seizures
	Theophylline (1)	Asthma
	Warfarin (Coumadin)	Blood-clotting problems
Pantoprazole	Digoxin (Lanoxin)	Heart disease
	Ketoconazole (Nizoral)	Fungal infection

(continued)

Table 10-5 *(continued)*

This Heartburn/ Reflux Drug	Interacts with: Generic Name (Brand Name)	Used to Treat This Condition
Rabeprazole	Diazapam (Valium)	Anxiety
	Digoxin (Lanoxin)	Heart disease
	Ketoconazole (Nizoral)	Fungal infection

* Many drugs are sold under several different brand names; this table lists one well-known one for each drug.
(1) This drug is most commonly prescribed as a generic.
(2) Other drugs in this class include amoxapine (Ascendin), nortriptyline (Aventyl), and imipramine (Tofranil).
(3) This class of drugs includes nicardipine (Cardene), diltiazem (Cardizem), amlodipine (Norvasc), and nifedipine (Procardia).
Sources: *Gastrogram: Spring 2001 (UHIC: Protein Pump Inhibitors...An Update);* The Handbook of Nonprescription Drugs, *13th ed. (Washington, D.C.: American Pharmaceutical Association, 2002);* Physicians' Desk Reference, *55th ed. (Montvale, N.J.: Medical Economics Company, 2001); Bruce T. Vanderhoff, Rundsarah M. Tahboub, "Proton Pump Inhibitors: An Update,"* American Family Physician, *July 15, 2002.*

Inviting your help on heartburn/reflux

The International Foundation for Functional Gastrointestinal Disorders (IFFGD) wants you! From time to time, IFFGD runs surveys designed to discover more information about people with gastrointestinal disorders including heartburn/reflux. The data from these surveys may help gastro researchers figure out how to make it easier for millions of people like you to treat and/or live with gastrointestinal problems including heartburn/reflux.

Of course, no one will know your name or contact you without your permission. So put on your mask, turn on your computer, and click to www.iffgd.org/Research/SurveyInvite.html for more information.

Chapter 11

Avoiding Problem Pills

. . . .

In This Chapter

▶ Describing how medicines may trigger reflux

▶ Loosening the LES

▶ Slowing the stomach

▶ Irritating the esophagus

▶ Taking meds safely

. . . .

*I*nteractions, adverse effects, and side effects are medicine's dirty little secrets. Pick a pill, any one at all, and darned if you can't find some problems hiding in the patient package insert.

If you actually take a few moments and read that handy-dandy little brochure, you can see that upset stomach is usually listed high as a common side effect. Reflux and heartburn aren't, but they should be.

This cautionary chapter alerts you to pharmaceutical troublemakers that may trigger reflux, make heartburn worse, or irritate delicate esophageal tissues. And, last but certainly not least, you can find some sensible strategies for taking your medicine without setting off a five-alarm case of heartburn. Who would expect anything less from a practical *For Dummies* book?

Pinpointing Potential Problems

Imagine that you have a medical problem. You go to your doctor who says, "No big deal," and scribbles off a prescription. You fill the prescription, take the medicine, and then, wow! you've got the Mother of All Heartburn. What in the world is happening?

As your doctor said, it's no big deal — to explain, that is. A medicine that gives you heartburn is doing one (or more) of the following unpleasant things to your gut:

✔ Loosening your lower esophageal sphincter (LES), so that acidic stomach contents back up into your esophagus. A weakened LES is almost certainly the most important cause of reflux. (For a complete explanation of what the LES is and its role in heartburn, check out Chapter 2.)

✔ Delaying the exit of food from your stomach, so that your full stomach presses up against your LES causing reflux, which causes heartburn.

✔ Irritating the delicate tissues of your esophagus.

If the problem persists, you may need to adapt your medicine to your heartburn. But not without reading the following warning (and the rest of this chapter).

If the medicine that seems to give you heartburn or make your heartburn worse is a *maintenance drug,* one you take regularly for a chronic condition (one example is insulin, which people with diabetes take on a regular schedule), then listen up: Don't change your dosage or stop taking this drug without first talking to your doctor.

Naming Medicines That Loosen the LES

Although I use the letters *LES* and the phrases *lower esophageal sphincter* and *loosen the LES* frequently enough to make you wish you'd never heard of them, you really do need to know that anything that relaxes the LES (the muscular trapdoor between the stomach and esophagus) increases the risk of acidic stomach contents flowing back into your esophagus.

Here's another mention of the LES. This time, I tell you that among the many things that trigger a loose LES are the many truly valuable medicines you may take on a daily basis, including those on the following, selected list. The medicines in this section directly weaken the LES.

When in doubt, check with your doctor. You can also spring for a copy of *The Essential Guide to Prescription Drugs 2004* by James J. Rybacki (Harper-Resources), a perfectly wonderful book that explains all about your medicines in terms an intelligent human being, such as you, can appreciate. (After you read it, check with your doctor, anyway!)

Antiasthma drugs

The characteristic symptom of asthma is *bronchial spasm,* a constriction of the tubes through which air flows in and out of your lungs. *Antiasthmatics* keep the tubes open.

The best-known antiasthma drug, *theophylline,* which just happens to be the primary stimulant in plain old tea, loosens the LES. Coffee also has theophylline, but java's most important stimulant is the related compound, caffeine, another LES loosener. Yes, both coffee and tea may loosen the LES.

Anticholinergics

Mammals, including human beings, have two kinds of nerves. The first type controls the muscles that actually move your various body parts. So long as you're healthy, you can move your arms and legs at will.

Another set of nerves comprise the *autonomic nervous system,* which does its work automatically. These nerves control such basic body functions such as

- ✔ Breathing
- ✔ Digesting
- ✔ Perspiring
- ✔ Salivating
- ✔ Secreting hormones

Anticholinergic drugs, such as antihistamines and antinausea meds, interrupt the activity of the autonomic nervous systems, including the nerves that open and close the LES. And when those nerves don't work at top efficiency, the risk of reflux rises.

Antidepressants

Tricyclic antidepressants, such as amitriptyline (Elavil), doxepin (Adapin), imipramine (Tofranil), and nortriptyline (Aventil), may benefit your psyche, but they may loosen the LES. Darn! That's depressing.

Antihypertensives

Do you have high blood pressure you can't lower with diet and exercise? Your doctor is likely to prescribe one of three types of meds:

- *Beta blockers,* such as atenolol (Tenormin), metoprolol (Toprol), and propranolol (Inderal), reduce the force with which your heart pumps blood out into your arteries.

- *Calcium channel blockers,* such as amlodipine (Norvasc), diltiazem (Cardizem), felodipine (Plendil), and nifedipine (Procardia), help keep your blood vessels relaxed and dilated wide enough to accommodate a free flow of blood.

- *Diurectics,* such as furosemide (Lasix), increase urination and reduce the amount of liquids in your body.

Beta blockers and calcium channel blockers may also (surprise) make the LES looser. (See the "What does a beta blocker block? What sails through a calcium channel?" sidebar in this chapter for more info on these types of high blood pressure meds.)

What does a beta blocker block? What sails through a calcium channel?

The quick answers: Beta blockers block the activity of beta-adrenergic receptors, and calcium channels are pathways for calcium molecules. Which raises two more questions. First, what are the first receptor thingees? Second, why wouldn't a person want to pack as much calcium as possible through those channels?

Beta-adrenergic receptors are specialized cells in your heart, kidneys, lungs, uterus, liver, and blood vessels, and adipose (fatty) tissue regulates reactions such as the speed at which your heart beats or the strength with which the smooth muscles such as those lining the uterus and blood vessels contract. The drugs called beta blockers block these reactions and may, for example, slow down an abnormally fast heartbeat, relax blood vessels to bring high blood pressure down, or weaken uterine muscle contractions to slow down premature labor.

Calcium channels are passages through which molecules of calcium (yes, the mineral) enter each body cell, which is good. Your body can't work without calcium. On the other hand, activated calcium channels lead to the contraction of blood vessels. Overly active calcium channels can actually constrict blood vessels to the point where too little blood reaches important muscles, such as your heart. Calcium channel blockers are medicines that reduce the flow of calcium, thus alleviating *angina* (pain in the heart muscles).

Anti-Parkinson medication

Levodopa (Dopar, Larodopa) is one the best-known members of a class of drugs that control the involuntary tremors (shaking) of Parkinson disease. These drugs may — yes, you're right! — loosen the LES.

Female hormones

Is there anything wider than the big, wide world of women's hormones? Hormones for birth control, hormones for menstrual distress, hormones for menopause — where does it end? Unfortunately, right back at the juncture between your stomach and your esophagus, your old familiar LES.

Women who have used oral contraceptives know from experience that the Pill can cause tummy tumult. Now, scientists from the Karolinska Institute in Stockholm concur about hormones used to relieve menopausal discomfort, either HRT (a combination of estrogen and progesterone) or estrogen alone.

The Karolinska study drew data from more than 60,000 Norwegian men and women. You can put the info on men aside right now; it talks about the effects of overweight on the risk of reflux and you can read about that in Chapter 4. But the study also had some intriguing info on female hormones and reflux.

- As a rule, premenopausal women (with normal levels of estrogen) are more likely to experience heartburn than are women who have gone through menopause.

- Postmenopausal women who use hormone replacement therapy (HRT) (estrogen plus progestins) are more likely than women who never use hormones to develop reflux.

- Postmenopausal women who use estrogen alone are more than twice as likely as women who never used hormones to develop reflux.

- In a second study, obese women taking estrogen alone are 33 times more likely than women of normal weight who did not use hormones to end up with reflux. What's obese? Check that out in Chapter 13.

Scientists need to confirm the institute's research with more studies, but given the continuing controversy over the safety of hormone-replacement therapy, the Karolinska numbers may be the scientific equivalent of a hot flash.

Narcotics

Narcotics are very strong pain medicine. When used properly, under a doctor's direction, they can revolutionize pain control, making it possible for people to survive the agony of chronic illness, serious injury, and invasive surgery.

To patch or not to patch? A tale of two studies

Smoking is unequivocally linked to an increased risk of reflux. But how about trying to stop smoking? You may not believe this statement, but your attempt to quit may also set your heartburn humming if you use a nicotine patch to quiet your cravings during the nasty first days of tobacco withdrawal.

This conclusion arises from a 1996 study of 20 hardy volunteers at the University of Louisville. During the study, researchers applied either a real nicotine patch or a look-alike patch to each volunteer's arm. Then the researchers inserted a small tube into each volunteer's esophagus to measure acid levels during a 48-hour period.

The results, published in the *American Journal of Gastroenterology,* showed that volunteers wearing the real nicotine patches ended up with more acid in the esophagus, and that the effect was most pronounced when the volunteers were lying down. In other words, if you're using a nicotine patch to help you stop smoking and you develop reflux, peel off the patch before you crawl into bed at night. Sounds sensible. Until the second study arrived in 1999.

The Louisville scientists wrote that although their 1996 study did show a link between nicotine patches and heartburn, it had a few teensy-weensy flaws in design, so they set up the 1999 study to get a more accurate picture.

In the first study, the scientists had included both smokers and nonsmokers instead of smokers alone or quitters alone. Second, the researchers didn't watch what the volunteers ate, meaning that some of the participants could have stuffed their faces with food and beverages known to trigger reflux. And finally, nobody checked to make sure none of the volunteers lit up.

So in 1999, the researchers enrolled 20 volunteers, all smokers, some wearing a nicotine patch, others, the look-alike patch with no nicotine. For three days, the Louisville researchers joined researchers from McNeil Consumer Products (which happens to make and sell nicotine patches) to observe the volunteers. In the end, the researchers found no "statistically significant" difference among the volunteers in terms of heartburn, chest pain, nausea, or difficulty swallowing.

Conclusion? If a person with reflux must choose between continuing to smoke or using the patch, the sensible choice seems to be to go with the patch — unless, of course, the researchers decide to do a follow-up study and find different results. ***Note:*** You can find a chart listing the various nicotine patches available in the United States and Canada in Chapter 14.

Next to this blessing, the discomfort of narcotic-related reflux may seem like small potatoes indeed. But I still have to mention that some narcotics, including meperidine (Demerol), may loosen your LES. On the other hand, doctors usually prescribe narcotics for short-term therapy, so the reflux may also be short term and the risk of addiction to a strong painkiller is minimized.

Nitrates

Angina is chest pain caused by reduced blood flow due to temporary constriction of the constricted blood vessels supplying your heart. *Nitrates* are drugs that relax blood vessels and improve blood flow to your heart, thus alleviating the pain of chronic angina.

The best-known nitrate is *nitroglycerin.* Like others in its class, such as isosorbide mononitrate, nitroglycerin may — surprise, surprise — loosen the LES. (You knew I was going to say that, didn't you?)

Sedatives and tranquilizers

Diazepam (Valium) and other short-term antianxiety drugs do a super job of relieving anxiety — except, perhaps, the anxiety linked to the loosey-goosey LES that may follow your taking these drugs.

Targeting Traffic Stoppers

A weakened LES is almost certainly the most important cause of reflux. The medicines listed in the "Naming Medicines That Loosen the LES" section directly weaken the LES. Many of them raise your risk of reflux in a second way, by slowing the exit of food from your stomach.

The longer the food you eat hangs around in your stomach, the longer your full stomach pushes up against the LES, raising your reflux risk.

For example, earlier in this chapter, you can read how anticholinergic drugs interrupt or slow the action of the autonomic nervous system. Well, that just happens to be the group of nerves that control *peristalsis,* the muscular contractions of the walls of the digestive tube. Peristalsis propels food from the stomach to the small intestine, then on to the large intestine, and finally out of your body. Weaken the peristaltic contractions and your stomach doesn't empty as quickly as it should, meaning you're in trouble.

In addition to anticholinergics, the drugs that slow peristalsis include

- ✔ Antianxiety medicine
- ✔ Narcotics
- ✔ Sedatives
- ✔ Tranquilizers

On the other hand, these two-problems-in-one-product medicines don't usually irritate your esophageal lining. That's a job for the drugs listed in the next section.

Listing Irritating Drugs and Supplements

Your stomach's lining is designed to resist the damaging effects of stomach acid, a logical situation considering that you need the acid to digest the food you swallow. But your esophageal lining isn't so lucky. This slippery tissue is designed to speed food down the food tube to your stomach, not to digest it on the way. As a result, when the acidic stomach contents reflux back through an open LES, the esophageal lining suffers. If you listen carefully, you may even hear it yelling, "Help!"

You may not always feel the acids eating away at your esophagus, but the more persistent your reflux and the longer you live with it, the more serious the damage done by stomach acids may be. In some cases, the injury is severe enough to cause *Barrett's esophagus,* a precancerous change in cells lining the esophagus. In worse cases, the changes proceed to esophageal cancer.

Your heartburn may have already damaged your esophagus, so you need to be especially aware of drugs and conditions that can do further damage. In this section I give you the scoop on some of these drugs — along with a word on some of the drugs that irritate your esophagus and may also irritate your stomach.

Given the stomach's ability to stand up to the acid that wreaks havoc on your esophagus, you may be completely stunned to hear that some medicines can do the same kind of damage in your stomach. What? A stomach lining that secretes acids strong enough to digest everything from baked beans to bratwurst may be done in by one or two insignificant little pills? In a word, absolutely.

Although the damage to the stomach lining doesn't increase your risk of reflux or intensify the injury to the esophageal lining, it definitely adds to your general discomfort — which makes it worth mentioning here.

Analgesics

The nonsteroidal anti-inflammatory drugs (NSAIDs, pronounced *en*-seds) are a big family that includes aspirin, celecoxib (Celebrex), ibuprofen (Advil, Motrin), naproxen (Aleve, Anaprox, Naprosyn), and rofecoxib (Vioxx). These valuable pain relievers are infamous for their ability to irritate the stomach lining, sometimes to the point of persistent bleeding, ulcer, or even hemorrhage.

And did I mention they may also have two other effects? They may upset your stomach, and they may increase your risk of reflux. Although everyone experiences some irritation when taking an NSAID, not everybody experiences reflux. If you do experience reflux while taking one of these drugs, ask your doctor to help you switch to a different NSAID; one may prove less upsetting than another. Or you may get relief by changing to acetaminophen (Tylenol), which is kinder to the stomach but doesn't have the NSAIDs' ability to reduce inflammation.

But as usual, things aren't always that simple. Because NSAIDs irritate the lining of the stomach, you may reasonably assume they would irritate the lining of the esophagus and increase the damage done by reflux. Surprise.

Recent studies have suggested that patients who take NSAIDs and aspirin are *less* likely to develop cell changes leading to esophageal cancer, and some researchers are using these medications to prevent worsening of patients with Barrett's esophagus (precancerous changes in esophageal tissues; see Chapter 4). Another reason to stay tuned — and to discuss all your medicines with your doctor.

Antibiotics

If you've ever taken azithromycin (Zithromax), clarithomycin (Biaxin), erythromycin (E-Mycin, Ilosone), or any tetracycline antibiotic, you probably know these pills can upset you stomach and increase your risk of reflux.

You probably also know then that if you follow the dosing instructions to the letter, including taking some antibiotics with food, that you may be able to make the side effects less annoying. But taking antibiotics with food isn't always the best way to go, so be sure to ask your doctor before you doctor up the way you take your meds.

Bone builders

Your body destroys old bone cells and builds new ones every day. This natural process is conducted by *osteoclasts* (the terminators) and *osteoblasts* (the builders). As you age, the former keep on truckin', but the latter slow down a bit. Older folks don't build new bone as fast as they destroy old bone, and the inevitable result is *osteoporosis,* a weakening of the bone that increases the risk of fractures.

Alendronate (Fosamax) and risedronate (Actonel) are *bisphosphonates,* compounds that inhibit osteoclasts from munching away on old bone, thus preserving what you already have, while osteoblasts build new bone.

Alas, as is so often the case in medicine, every bit of good news comes with a dash of not-so-good news. No surprise here: Bisphosphonates may irritate the esophagus.

You *may* be able to avoid this irritation if the pill passes quickly into your stomach. Proposed solution: Take your meds in the morning, on an empty stomach, with a full glass of water, and stay upright — no crawling back into bed for a snooze — for at least 30 minutes.

Other esophagus irritators

If you don't take your pill with a glass of water, it may stick to the side of the esophagus; in extreme cases, this may damage the esophageal lining. Some medicines, however, may be irritating even if you take them correctly:

- ✔ Quinidine (Cardioquin, Duraquin), a drug to control irregular heartbeat
- ✔ Tetracycline derivatives, antibiotics to control infection

If you're taking any of these meds, make sure you take them with plenty of water. If you develop painful swallowing or find it hard to move food down the esophagus, call your doctor right away.

Nutritional supplements

Some common supplements seem to see your stomach (and your esophagus) as a challenge. Pop a vitamin C, iron, or potassium pill into your mouth and as it slides down your gullet, the little bugger is thinking, "Boy, oh, boy, what trouble can I cause today?"

Both vitamin C and iron can upset your stomach and irritate your esophagus. To counter their natural inclination to be troublesome,

- ✔ Stick to a reasonable dose (2,000 mg vitamin C is more irritating than 100 mg).
- ✔ Take the pill with food and water.

For more about vitamins, minerals and other nutritional supplements, check out Chapter 5.

Naming Medical Conditions That May Make Meds Stick

Do you have trouble swallowing hard drugs? No, not that kind of hard drugs. I mean *pills, tablets,* and *capsules.* If so, your medicine may stick to the side of your esophagus, an uncomfortable, even painful, situation that can irritate the esophageal lining. This problem is most likely to occur among people who have the following medical conditions:

- ✔ *Achalasia,* a fancy way of saying that their esophageal muscles contract weakly or irregularly, slowing the movement of food — and pill — from mouth to stomach.
- ✔ Esophageal spasms, a muscle contraction that may suddenly narrow the esophagus, stopping the food — or pill — right in its tracks.
- ✔ Esophageal *stricture,* a physical narrowing of the tube caused by previous damage to the tissues. The narrowing naturally interferes with the free flow of food — or pill.

In each case, the result may be a pill that stays in your esophagus, irritating the tissues, sometimes enough to cause bleeding, perforation (a hole in the wall), or a stricture.

You may be able to ease a pill's passage by taking your medicine with a full glass of water. But achalasia, spasms, and stricture are real medical conditions. Check with your doctor before pouring on the water. The better solution may be a different form of the drug.

Difficulty in swallowing is a warning sign of gastroesophageal reflux disease (GERD). If you experience problems swallowing food or liquids, run, don't walk, to your doctor.

Minimizing the Heartburn Effects of Essential Medicines

In this fun part, I get to list rules to reduce the risk of reflux posed by problem pills. Of course, these rules are pretty fundamental and I bet you've seen them a dozen times before, but repetition makes remembering them easier.

Read the label

As you read the label on your medicine, check out several important pieces of information to make sure you have the correct prescription. Check

- The drug's name
- The dose
- The doctor's name
- The patient's name (yes, it's your name)

What? It's not your name? If it isn't, forget about reflux risk. Just take those pills right back to the drugstore and get the correct prescription.

Don't chew the pills

If the direction says, "Take this tablet whole," then don't chew the pill. Don't crush it either. Many common pills have an *enteric coating,* a special covering that protects the pill from stomach acid so it passes unscathed through your stomach to dissolve in your small intestine. Other pills may be rendered ineffective by stomach acid; a time-release pill could be made dangerously stronger if you release the ingredients all at once.

By the way, if the label on your pill bottle says "chewable" — usually in big letters — you can forget this rule. Remember there's an exception to every rule.

Don't take your pill lying down

Your aim is to get your medicine from your mouth to your stomach as quickly and smoothly as possible and keep it there. To do that, you need to maintain a straight downward path from your mouth to your esophagus through the junction where your esophagus meets your stomach.

As you can see in Figure 11-1, the best way to accomplish this goal is to sit up straight or stand up while taking your pill. If you lie down, the pill may easily slide back from your stomach to your esophagus, especially if you have a floppy LES. Even if your head hurts like crazy, sit up, take your meds, and stay upright for several minutes.

And, yes, an exception exists here. If your prescription says "Sit up for 30 minutes after taking this medicine" (see "Bone builders" in this chapter), then sit up. And consider the fact that the only way to take your meds safely and effectively is to read the label first, even if it means hauling out a magnifying glass to read the tiny type.

Don't forget the water

Taking your pill with a full glass of plain water helps move the pill swiftly through your esophagus to your stomach. No sticking to the esophageal lining equals less risk of irritation.

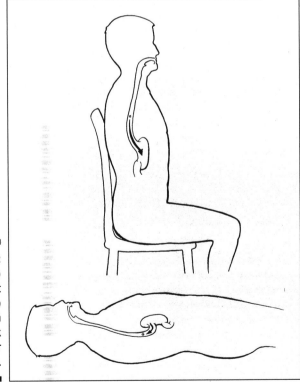

Figure 11-1:
Sitting up straight helps keep pills from sliding back into your esophagus.

Why water? Because plain water — no bubbles, please — doesn't make you burp, as soft drinks may. Plain water is calorie-free, so it doesn't add pounds. Milk's drawback is that it interacts with some meds; tea and coffee are hot, so you can't drink 'em down right away. Yep, plain water's best.

Eat a little

If the label says "take this medication with food," it means either that the medicine is more effective if you have food in your stomach or that having food in your stomach when you swallow the pill reduces the risk of gastric upset, thus lowering the risk of reflux and protecting your esophagus.

The flip side: If the label says "take this pill on an empty stomach," you should. Sometimes having food in your stomach interferes with the drug's ability to dissolve and get to the body part it's meant to treat.

Chapter 12

Exploring Surgical Options

. . . .

In This Chapter

▶ Selecting the appropriate candidates for surgery

▶ Explaining the operation

▶ Evaluating the results

▶ Going home

▶ Looking at the future

. . . .

*R*ight off the bat, you should know that heartburn surgery is a controversial subject. After all, up to 90 percent of people with heartburn/reflux feel better after simply avoiding annoying foods, giving up tobacco, controlling their weight, or taking the appropriate medicine.

For the very small group of patients whose severe reflux doesn't respond to these easy remedies, surgery may be an option. But the operative — yes, it's a terrible pun — word in the sentence is *may*. Most heartburn experts agree that heartburn surgery is almost always an elective procedure. Virtually no one *has* to have it. As a result, deciding who may benefit from the procedure is a complicated procedure in its own right.

Frankly speaking, if your reflux responds to diet, meds, or changes in your lifestyle, you probably have better things to do than read this chapter. If you do read it, keep in mind that it comes with a warning label: What you're about to read is for information only. Your doctor, the person most familiar with your medical history, is the only one who may recommend surgical treatment — the procedure known as fundoplication, which I cover a bit later in this chapter.

Nominating Candidates for Heartburn Surgery

This election is one nobody really wants to win. Although this operation is sometimes called *heartburn surgery,* the procedure isn't for people with an occasional twinge in the esophagus or even those who have reflux fewer than two or three times a week.

You don't even have to think about the surgical option for snuffing out that heartburn until you've tried the other tried-and-true measures I discuss elsewhere in this book:

- ✔ Changing your diet to avoid irritating foods and beverages (more about that in Chapter 6)

- ✔ Finding a more comfortable way to sleep (Chapter 16)

- ✔ Giving up cigarettes and reducing your consumption of alcohol (Chapter 14)

- ✔ Losing weight to reduce the pressure on your esophagus (Chapter 13)

- ✔ Taking medicines to neutralize or reduce the acid refluxing from your stomach (more about that in Chapter 10)

If none of these approaches has succeeded in extinguishing the fire in your esophagus, the word *surgery* — or the more modern term *surgical procedure* — may suddenly float into the air in your doctor's office. Don't panic. Before your doctor zips you off to be unzipped, you have to pass (fail?) a number of medical tests to prove you're a good surgical candidate.

Figuring out who actually is a candidate for surgery requires evaluating your symptoms and the condition of your esophagus. Your first step, therefore, is to find the right doctor. In this case, you're looking for a *gastroenterologist,* a doctor specializing in disorders of the digestive tract such as reflux. The gastroenterologist may also be a surgeon, but you never go straight from your primary care physician's (PCP's) office to the operating table. Your PCP is the gatekeeper, but the person who unlocks the door should be a specialist. (I cover the ins and outs of finding the right doctor in Chapter 8.)

Meeting medication malcontents

A number of medication-related issues could signal surgical considerations:

✔ **Continuing symptoms:** Although reflux medications provide relief for most people with heartburn, some patients still have symptoms even when taking medicine. The symptoms may be due to reflux, or to some other medical condition such as a pulmonary infection or a respiratory allergy. If reflux is to blame, surgery may be an option. How can you place the blame squarely on the shoulders of reflux? With the tests I cover in Chapter 9.

✔ **Strong aversion to pills:** Surgery may also be an option for people who really hate taking pills. (You conveniently "forget" to swallow one a day and/or you can't stand the thought of taking a pill a day forever and ever.) Sound familiar?

Wait! Is the one thing sending you to surgery your refusal to take a daily pill? Then you may want to think about sitting down with an appropriate therapist to work out your aversion to medicine. No surgery is risk-free. In the absence of unbearable side effects, you can see that taking heartburn pills is less potentially injurious than an operation. And it's such a teensy little pill. Think about it.

✔ **Related side effects:** Like other medicines, antireflux medicines do come with some — mostly mild — adverse effects. Like what? You may experience

- Abdominal pain
- Breast tenderness
- Constipation
- Impotence
- Nausea
- Headache

Ordinarily, these symptoms aren't likely to be debilitating, but everyone is different, and if your drug side effects are so unpleasant that you regularly experience the desire to flush the pills, surgery may seem reasonable.

Assessing esophagus damage

Continuing exposure to acid liquids bouncing up from your stomach may seriously damage or erode the lining of the esophagus. In the worst-case scenario, the damage may lead to esophageal cancer. If your reflux is injuring your esophagus badly enough to raise your risk of cancer, surgery may be an option to consider.

Before recommending surgery, your doctor will want to know if your reflux is severe enough to damage the lining of your esophagus *or* whether your esophageal lining already shows the wounds typical of erosion or the cellular changes that predict cancer. To find out, she can order one or more of the series of diagnostic tests that I describe in Chapter 9. The four tests she is most likely to choose are

- **24-hour pH study:** During this test, your doctor puts a very small tube into your esophagus to collect samples of the liquid in your throat during a 24-hour period in order to measure the local acidity. If the acidity is higher than normal, your doctor may select surgery to reduce your exposure to reflux, which will damage your esophagus.

- **Barium swallow:** For this test, you swallow a thick solution containing the element barium that coats your esophagus's lining. An X-ray examination shows any abnormalities, such as a narrowed esophagus or ulcers, outlined by the barium.

- **Esophageal manometry:** To perform this test, your doctor threads a thin, flexible tube through your nose into your esophagus and stomach to measure the pressure in your esophagus and the strength of your esophageal muscles. By doing so, your doctor can decide whether you have the muscle power required to push food through the surgically tightened opening between your esophagus and stomach.

- **Upper endoscopy:** This test gives doctor an up-close-and-personal picture of your esophageal lining via a small viewing tube/camera in your throat. Your doctor can see obvious erosion of the tissue through the camera. If she finds sites suggestive of precancerous changes, she'll remove small tissue samples to evaluate changes in the cells, a procedure called a *biopsy.*

Stop! Don't run away! Yes, these tests sound miserable, and no, they aren't a walk in the park. But proper anesthesia can alleviate the discomfort and make them bearable.

Considering other factors

You want to consider other important factors when evaluating your need for heartburn surgery, such as the state of your

- **Hiatus:** If you have a large *hiatal hernia* (a gap in the muscle around the place where the esophagus meets the stomach), surgery may offer a cure for your reflux, but having a hiatal hernia doesn't mean you have to have surgery.

- **Health:** If you have asthma, or you experience hoarseness or coughing that hangs around even when you're taking heartburn meds, you may want to consider surgery, but only after ruling out a respiratory problem that can be treated and/or cured with another method. What other method? Antibiotics for an infection or antihistamines for seasonal allergies come quickly to mind.

Are you beginning to feel a push/pull at work here? Remember, this is a controversial subject because most people with heartburn feel better with simple changes in diet as I outline in Chapter 6 or with the antireflux medicines I describe in Chapter 10.

Taking the surgery option off the table

Heartburn surgery may be off the table (operating table, that is) for these types of patients:

- ✔ **An older adult in poor health:** As life expectancy lengthens, the definition of "old" has changed, so that you have to be in your 80s before you qualify as "old." At the same time, advances in anesthesia and surgical techniques have pushed the treatment envelope way back for aging patients who are now routinely offered treatment as aggressive as that prescribed for their kids and grandkids.

  The accepted exception for surgery may be an elderly person with a long list of health problems, such as heart disease or circulation or breathing problems, which may be complicated by anesthesia and surgical injury. But consider the word *may*. The one immutable fact of modern medicine is — you never know.

- ✔ **An esophageal weakling:** People whose esophageal muscles are so weak that they have trouble pushing foods down through the esophagus may be worse off with a tight LES. As I note earlier in the chapter, smart doctors test esophageal muscle strength before recommending heartburn surgery.

Setting a Surgical Schedule

If your gastroenterologist believes that surgery can help relieve your gastroesophageal reflux disease (GERD), the next move is to find a surgeon who performs heartburn surgery. Sometimes you don't have to look very far. Your gastroenterologist may be a surgeon. If not, he's likely to recommend a surgeon he knows and trusts. Because heartburn surgery is elective surgery, you should have the time to check out his choice and make sure you're comfortable with the new doctor.

Selecting a surgeon

One good guide to choosing a surgeon is Chapter 8, which lays out some basic rules for finding and choosing any doctor. In medicine, as in other fields, practice makes perfect — or at least *more skilled*. The more procedures a doctor has performed, the better your chances for a successful outcome. How many is *more?* Experts put the bottom line for heartburn surgery at around 50 operations.

Because you're talking surgery, which requires that you spend some time in a hospital, in addition to being comfortable with your choice of surgeon, you want to know what hospital the surgeon uses and how familiar he is with the surgery you're about to have. More experience is also assumed to be better for hospitals. An institution where the doctors, nurses, and anesthesiologists perform tons of heartburn surgery is a place where people tend to know the ins and outs of the operation (not to mention the sometimes-surprising little glitches that may arise when one human being cuts into another). One way to find an area hospital that has performed a bunch of heartburn surgeries is to click on www.google.com and type "fundoplication rates [your city] hospitals". The information you get varies from city to city, but this search phrase is a good starting point.

Prepping for surgery

The tests are done. You've met with your surgeon who says, "Let's go with the surgery." You're on your way. But where are you going?

For most people, the days or weeks between "Let's go" and "Scalpel, please" often seem like a mystical medical maze. Being nervous is completely normal at this time. But to avoid feeling totally overwhelmed, sit quietly and calmly — yes, calmly — and consider the schedule ahead of you.

The first step: Your doctor must pick a date for the operation. After that, her nurse/assistant/patient specialist can

✔ Schedule you for pre-admittance blood tests.

✔ Schedule an interview with an anesthesiologist. (***Note:*** This interview may occur in the hospital right before surgery.)

✔ Give you a printed sheet with instructions and the important dates. *Don't leave your doctor's office without this incredibly important piece of paper.* When you're stressed — like when your doctor has just scheduled you for surgery — your memory is unreliable. The paperwork the folks at the doc's office will give you tells you when and where to arrive for surgery and how to prepare, for example, by avoiding all food and beverages for 12 hours before surgery.

When the big day comes, and you're sitting there hungry, thirsty, and in a gown that doesn't quite close in the back . . . just close your eyes. Think good thoughts and try to relax. The next few hours belong to your surgeon — remember he's an expert.

Cutting and Pasting: Fundoplication

No matter what chapter you read first in this book, you're going to run into a paragraph describing the function (and misfunction) of the *lower esophageal sphincter*. This valve, also known as the LES, is the trapdoor between your esophagus and your stomach. Your LES closes tight after you swallow to prevent acidic stomach contents from sliding back — or refluxing — into your esophagus.

Rudolf Nissen, 1898–1981

In 1930, when Rudolf Nissen was appointed professor of medicine at the prestigious Berlin Charite hospital, his future seemed assured. But with Adolph Hitler's rise to power in 1933, "non-Aryan" professionals such as Nissen were forced out of their jobs, out of their homes, and often to their deaths.

Nissen was one of those lucky enough to escape. Pretending to be going on vacation, he and his wife fled to Switzerland, hoping to make that the first stop on their way to the United States. But after he and his wife were across the Swiss border, Nissen received an invitation from the Turkish government to join the faculty at the University of Istanbul. He accepted and went on to serve as surgeon and teacher in Istanbul until 1937. Then, as Turkey and Germany became allies heading into the Second World War, he was once again forced to flee.

This time, Nissen did reach the United States, one in a wave of thousands of German refugees, including such intellectual leaders as Albert Einstein (a Nissen patient), artists Max Ernst and Marc Chagall, and architect Ludwig Mies van der Rohe. Within two years, working as a research assistant in Boston, Nissen had mastered English and was invited to resume his surgical career, this time in Brooklyn, New York, where he joined the Jewish Hospital (today known as Interfaith Medical Center) and Maimonides Medical Center, while serving as associate professor at the Long Island College of Medicine.

At the war's end, the Berlin Charite sought to make amends by inviting Nissen to return. He refused, preferring instead to go back to Switzerland in 1951 as chairman of the Department of Surgery at the University of Basel. In ensuing years, he perfected a number of techniques for esophageal surgery including, of course, the Nissen fundoplication. In 1966, the year before he retired, Nissen finally accepted an honorary doctorate from Berlin's Humboldt University.

The most common cause of reflux leading to heartburn is a floppy LES. So don't be surprised to hear that heartburn surgery is designed to tighten the area around the LES, enabling the trapdoor to stay protectively shut after you've swallowed your food.

Medical textbooks and dictionaries are full of conditions, organs, and procedures named for the people who identified, discovered, or invented them. The surgery for heartburn is called *fundoplication*. The first, most basic form of this operation is the Nissen fundoplication, the procedure invented in 1951 by Rudolf Nissen — which is why it's called the *Nissen fundoplication* instead of, say, the Smith fundoplication.

The Nissen fundoplication is the surgical gold standard for people with GERD. In this fold-and-stitch procedure, your surgeon folds the top of your stomach around the base of your esophagus, thus tightening the area around the LES. After surgery, the wrap helps keep the LES closed, preventing reflux even when you've eaten and your stomach is full.

Not simple enough? Well, as some smart cookie once said: "One picture is worth a thousand words." So for your viewing pleasure, Figure 12-1 offers not one, not two, but three clear pictures to help you see how the Nissen fundoplication narrows the esophagus.

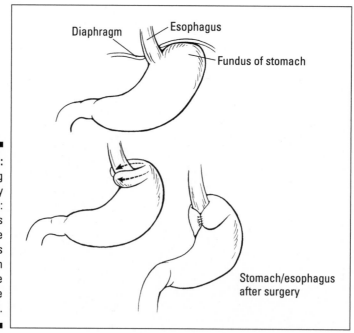

Figure 12-1:
Folding away heartburn: The fundus of the stomach is drawn around the base of the esophagus.

Diaphragm — Esophagus

Fundus of stomach

Stomach/esophagus after surgery

Your doctor can also use fundoplication to repair a hiatal hernia. When you have a hiatal hernia, your stomach pushes up through the opening in your diaphragm, creating pressure in the LES, which can pop up to permit reflux. (For more about hiatal hernias and their role in reflux, check out Chapter 4.)

Opening moves

For four decades, from the time Rudolf Nissen created the procedure in 1951, fundoplication was performed as "open" surgery. Translation: Through a relatively large (6- to 8-inch) incision.

Then in 1991, surgeons working in Belgium and the United States introduced newer, less traumatic laparoscopic methods. Now, instead of cutting one long incision, a surgeon performing laparoscopic fundoplication can

✔ Make four or five small incisions into the abdomen

✔ Insert a *trocar* (a thin tube) into each incision

✔ Thread a *laparoscope* (a small viewing scope attached to a TV camera) through one trocar to broadcast a closed-circuit picture of your insides

✔ Insert four additional trocars to accommodate the special surgical instruments used to perform the procedure

Figure 12-2 shows the placement of the incisions for laparoscopic fundoplication. To visualize the incision for open fundoplication, just connect the dots, um, incisions.

Figure 12-2:
Surgical incisions for laparoscopic Nissen fundoplication.

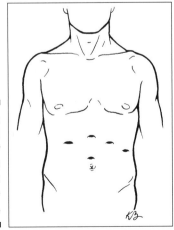

Fundoplication? What kind of word is that?

The term *fundoplication* is nothing more than a combination of two words that spell relief for people with heartburn. Fundoplication, pronounced fun-*do*-plih-*kay*-shun, begins with fundo = *fundus* = the top of the stomach, and pairs that with -plication = *plica,* Latin for *folded,* to make a word that means "folding the top of the stomach."

As you can see in Table 12-1, laparoscopic fundoplication offers several advantages over open surgery.

But — there's always a *but* — laparoscopy may not be the best choice for patients who have had previous abdominal surgery that left scar tissue, which complicates the new procedure. Your doctor, the person most familiar with your medical status, is the only one who knows for sure which path works best for you.

Table 12-1	Comparing Surgical Effects	
	From Open Surgery	*From Laparoscopy*
Incision	One 6–8 inch	Four to five 0.5–1 inch
Closing incision	Stitches	Tape
Pain level	Higher	Lower
Scar(s)	Long	Short
Days in hospital	4–7	1–2
Return to work	3–4 weeks	1 week
Time until full recovery	6 weeks	1–2 weeks

Working the inside track

Whether you and your surgeon choose open surgery or a laparoscopic surgery, the basic outline of the procedure is the same.

Playing the name game: Fundoplication variations

This sidebar contains descriptions from the National Institute of Diabetes and Digestive and Kidney Diseases' of the several variations on the basic fundoplication technique I describe in this chapter. For example, although each variety of fundoplication tightens the area of the LES to reduce the risk of reflux:

✔ The Nissen fundoplication folds the fundus completely around the base of the esophagus.

✔ The Toupet partial fundoplication wraps the fundus half way around the base of the esophagus.

✔ The Hill repair attaches the esophagus to the fundus rather than wrapping the fundus around the esophagus.

✔ The Belsey-Mark fundoplication wraps the fundus ⅔ of the way around the esophagus and stitches the wrap to the diaphragm.

Having opened you up, a lot or a little, your surgeon

1. Lifts (or nudges) aside your liver so he can clearly see your stomach's fundus.

2. Carefully cuts through the tissue attaching the fundus to your *spleen,* an organ sitting behind your stomach.

3. Draws the fundus forward and very gently wraps the fundus around the base of your esophagus, taking care to avoid internal bruising that may cause extra discomfort as you heal.

4. Stitches the folded stomach in place.

   Time out! If you have a hiatal hernia, your doctor repairs it now. Time in!

5. Closes the incision(s). He stitches an open incision; laparoscopic incisions are small enough to be taped shut.

And then you get a nice neat bandage and a fun ride on a rolling cart (gurney) off to the recovery room.

Meeting the Morning After

Your doctor has done the heavy lifting. Now the scalpels are back in the drawer, and you're back in the Land of the (semi) Conscious, ready to take command of your own recovery, or at least to begin to think about what comes next.

Returning to the real world

As your anesthesia wears off, and you blink open your baby blues, your first conscious thought is likely to be, "Hey that wasn't too bad."

You may find that your doctor left a tube in your nose that goes down to your stomach. The tube is a device to enable *any* air sitting around the surgical site at the bottom of your esophagus to escape easily, rather than hang around as uncomfortable bloat. (More about bloat in the "Floating on bloat" section, later in the chapter.)

Relieving your pain

Next surprise: No pain. Or practically none. Yes, small laparoscopic incisions are always less painful than long, open incisions, but either way, the nurse makes sure you have sufficient pain medication. If you hurt, don't be shy. Ask for more.

After surgery, some would-be Supermen and Wonder Women refuse to ask for pain meds because they fear becoming addicts. This superhero act is foolish bravado. When you hurt, all your systems go on alert, further stressing your already stressed body and slowing your recovery. In other words, *adequate pain relief is good medical practice.* If you hurt, ask for help. Your short-term relief is just that: short-term relief. Not the path to perdition.

Getting out

You may be thinking, "How soon can I get out of here?" If *here* means bed, the answer is, pretty soon. In fact, you're likely to be up and around lickety-split — like in a couple of hours. Standing and walking as soon as possible reduce the risk of complications such as blood clots.

If *here* means the hospital, the length of your stay varies with the procedure. After open surgery, your stay is commonly measured in days, as few as three or as many as six. With laparoscopic surgery, your stay may be measured in hours, like 36 to 48. Some people may even get to go home the same day of the surgery. Naturally, individual bodies react differently, so these timelines are only guidelines.

Eating again

Remember how hungry and thirsty you were when you arrived for your date with the surgeon? Remember how you promised yourself a gourmet meal afterward? Will you settle for a few sips of a clear liquid advancing to soft solid — think gelatin — before you go home? I thought so.

Because reflux is so often associated with food, you may be thinking that Jell-O is all you're going to get for a while. On the contrary, this is just the first meal on the first day. It's designed to prevent nausea while your stomach is still a bit jumpy from anesthesia and to avoid irritating your insides that are still a bit sore from surgery.

Reaching Home Base

You can't wait until you reach the comfort of your own home. Your own pillow. Your own bed. Your own food. Your own life. Enjoy every little detail but

- ✔ Don't do any heavy lifting.
- ✔ Don't chase the cat or the kids.
- ✔ Sleep when you're tired.
- ✔ Take it easy.

Even the healthiest body needs a week or two to bounce back fully from laparoscopic surgery and up to six weeks to recover from open surgery. In the interim, you may experience one or more of the following usual and expected reactions.

Swallowing hard

Some doctors say every fundoplication patient has difficulty swallowing food in the first few days or weeks after surgery. Others say the incidence of *dysphagia* (medical-speak for "swallowing problems") may be as low as one in every five patients.

Of course, if that *one* is *you,* the incidence is 100 percent, so you'll be pleased to hear that most people who experience swallowing problems after fundoplication have only minor discomfort for a short period of time.

A small percentage, however, may have long-term swallowing problems, a condition that may require *dilation* (stretching) of the esophagus or — more rarely — a second surgery. Notice all the "mays" in there? Remember that individual bodies differ, requiring different approaches.

Reprising reflux

After esophageal surgery, most patients take antireflux/antacid meds for a while to protect sensitive tissues. No big deal.

A small number of fundoplication patients get their reflux back shortly after surgery, usually with mild symptoms. An even smaller number may need a second surgery. Finally, over time, the repair may break down. One study found two-thirds of surgery patients back on reflux medicines around ten years after the surgery.

Floating on bloat

Fundoplication tightens the LES, which means you may have to swallow harder to get food through. However, if you're swallowing harder, you're probably swallowing more air. Eventually, you'll swallow normally and gulp less air, but for now, you probably have more gas. Okay, so you just belch it up, right? Not exactly. Immediately after surgery, you may have trouble burping. As a result, your gas hangs around, and you feel bloated and uncomfortable.

Eating soft foods such as scrambled eggs or applesauce may relieve some of the bloating distress. Soft foods go down easier, so you don't have to push and you swallow less air. Eating more slowly is also a time-honored antigas stratagem.

If you're a dinner sprinter — a person who usually inhales a four-course meal in four minutes flat — stop. Slow down. Chew each mouthful 100 times. Okay, so just chew 50 times. Listen, even chewing your food a measly ten times before swallowing is better than bolting it whole. And doesn't food taste better when you give yourself some time to enjoy it? Yes.

Balancing Risks and Benefits

Why is this chapter so cautious about heartburn surgery? Because no surgery is completely risk-free. For example, fundoplication carries a low risk of death, estimated by the Mayo Clinic to be less than 1 in every 500 patients. Serious complications may occur in up to 4 of every 100 patients having laparoscopic fundoplication (the incidence is presumably higher among those having open surgery). The following list contains some potentially serious complications after surgery, several specific to fundoplication:

✔ A bad reaction to the anesthesia.

✔ Excess bleeding during or after surgery that may require a transfusion.

When your doctor schedules surgery, ask if you can arrange to donate your own blood to be stored for use —if needed — during your operation, thus reducing the risk of transfusion reactions.

✔ Accidental perforation of the stomach or esophagus.

✔ Infection of the wound that may cause pain and fever.

✔ Postsurgical pneumonia.

✔ Blood clots in the legs.

✔ Slippage in the wrap of the fundus (requires surgical repair).

✔ Slippage of the fundus up through the diaphragm into the chest (requires surgical repair).

Read this list carefully. But consider this fact carefully, too: When Mayo Clinic experts drafted this list, they also found that up to 98 percent of the people who have fundoplication were happy with the results a year later.

The point? If your reflux is serious enough to convince your doctor to recommend surgery, the benefits — no more pain, no more esophageal damage — are likely to outweigh the risks. The counterpoint? It's your body. Only you can make that choice.

Peering into the Reflux Crystal Ball

When predicting the future of treatment for heartburn and reflux, bulletins from the U.S. Food and Drug Administration (FDA) beat a crystal ball every time. Recently the FDA approved three interesting new surgical techniques.

The iffy cloud in the crystal ball shows that no long-term stats are currently available to prove the effectiveness of any of these three new techniques. But in a country with millions of reflux patients, you can certainly bet that gastro gurus here — and around the world — are eagerly waiting to see what time will tell.

Seeing future No .1

The Bard EndoCinch is a procedure during which the surgeon stitches tiny little pleats in the LES to strengthen the valve. This procedure seems to decrease reflux symptoms and has been approved for general use, although questions remain about its ability to control reflux for the long term. At least one other company is making and marketing a different "sewing machine" for reflux.

Seeing future No. 2

The Stretta system relies on an electrode to make tiny cuts in the surface of the LES, forming scar tissue intended to toughen the muscle. This system also has been demonstrated to control symptoms. Several significant side effects (including a couple of deaths) have been reported after use of this device, yet it continues to be used and studied.

Seeing future No. 3

Enteryx is a *polymer* (plastic) solution that is implanted into the wall of the lower esophagus. After the injection, the liquid in the solution passes down through the esophagus, leaving the polymer to solidify into a bouncy pad that may help keep your LES closed after you swallow. A short (12-month), small (85-patient) study showed that two-thirds stopped taking reflux medication entirely after an Enteryx implant. Another 9 percent cut the dose by at least half. The side effects were similar to those following fundoplication: temporary pain, difficulty swallowing, and gas. Scientists are also looking for and testing other substances that can be injected into the LES to reduce the risk of reflux.

Part IV
Creating a Comfortable Lifestyle

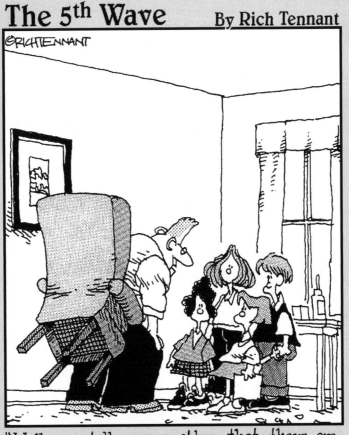

The 5th Wave   By Rich Tennant

"Well you tell your mother that there are no indications that I need to lose weight."

In this part . . .

Your general health, your good (and bad) habits, and — believe it or not — the clothes and makeup you wear and the furniture you sit and sleep on may all influence your heartburn. This part tells you how to adapt your daily living to reduce your reflux risk.

Chapter 13

Building a Better Body

*G*ot heartburn?

Unfortunately, you can't snap your fingers and alter your innards, particularly your lower esophageal sphincter (LES), but you can change the surrounding package in ways that may spell r-e-l-i-e-f. For example, losing a few pounds may reduce intestinal pressure leading to reflux, and a sensible exercise program may alleviate stress, another heartburn trigger.

Exercise and diet go hand in hand in making a slimmer, trimmer, healthier you, so this chapter tells you how to reach your goal by choosing a safe, effective diet and a workout plan that avoids common pitfalls.

Answering Question Numero Uno: Who's Overweight?

Carrying extra pounds can raise your risk of lots of medical problems including

- ✔ Arthritis
- ✔ Diabetes
- ✔ Heart disease

And yes, those extra pounds can increase the risks for heartburn. The mechanism is clear: Extra pounds around the middle press up against the lower part of your esophagus. The pressure increases the possibility that the LES, the opening between esophagus and stomach, will pop open, allowing acidic stomach contents to reflux back into the esophagus.

Is losing weight the answer? Maybe. But before you go on a weight-loss diet, take the time to be sure that you're carrying around more pounds than you should. How do you tell? Well, beauty may be in the eye of the beholder, but fat is in the Body Mass Index (BMI). BMI is a measurement introduced to the United States in 1990 by the National Heart, Lung, and Blood Institute (NHLBI), a member of the National Institutes of Health (NIH).

BMI is a unisex description of weight relative to height. The ratio is expressed in a number, such as 24, that serves as a predictor of your risk for weight-related illnesses, such as diabetes, high blood pressure, heart disease, stroke, gallbladder disease, and arthritic pain.

In the past decade, repeated studies have shown that BMI is a more accurate guide to who's overweight and to who's at risk of weight-related illness than simply jumping on the scale. In short, the higher your BMI, the higher your risk. So, cutting to the chase, what's your BMI?

Calculating your BMI

The original BMI equation was set up in kilograms for weight (W) and meters for height (H): BMI = W/H^2. If you live in Europe, Asia, or Canada, just plug in your very own personal metric numbers, such as 63.5 kilograms (kg) and 1.626 meters (m), and calculate away:

BMI = W/H^2 =

63.5 kilograms/(1.626 meters × 1.626 meters) =

63.5 kilograms/2.644 square meters =

24.01 BMI

Time out! Before I get to the mechanics of running the numbers for everyone in the states, you can sneak a peek at Table 13-1. Does a For Dummies book take care of you, or what? And, I guess if you really hate math, you can leave it at that. But, I'm assuming you're a curious kind of person like me who wants to know the story behind the numbers.

Table 13-1

Body Mass Index

Height (inches)	Body Weight (Pounds)																
	19	20	21	22	23	24	25	26	27	28	29	30	31	32	33	34	35
58	91	96	100	105	110	115	119	124	129	134	138	143	148	153	158	162	167
59	94	99	104	109	114	119	124	128	133	138	143	148	153	158	163	168	173
60	97	102	107	112	118	123	128	133	138	143	148	153	158	163	168	174	179
61	100	106	111	116	122	127	132	137	143	148	153	158	164	169	175	180	185
62	104	109	115	120	126	131	136	142	147	153	158	164	169	175	180	186	191
63	107	113	118	124	130	135	141	146	152	158	163	169	175	180	186	191	197
64	110	116	122	128	134	140	145	151	157	163	169	174	180	186	192	197	204
65	114	120	126	132	138	144	150	156	162	168	174	180	186	192	198	204	210
66	118	124	130	136	142	148	155	161	167	173	179	185	192	198	204	210	216
67	121	127	134	140	146	153	159	166	172	178	185	191	198	204	211	217	223
68	125	131	138	144	151	158	164	171	177	184	190	197	203	210	216	223	230
69	128	135	142	149	155	162	169	176	182	189	196	203	209	216	223	230	236
70	132	139	146	153	160	167	174	181	188	195	202	209	216	222	229	236	243
71	136	143	150	157	165	172	179	186	193	200	208	215	222	229	236	243	250
72	140	147	154	162	169	177	184	191	199	206	213	221	228	235	242	250	258
73	144	151	159	166	174	182	189	197	204	212	219	227	235	242	250	257	265
74	148	155	163	171	179	186	194	202	210	218	225	233	241	249	256	264	272
75	152	160	168	176	184	192	200	208	216	224	232	240	248	256	264	272	279
76	156	164	172	180	189	197	205	213	221	230	238	246	254	263	271	279	287

Source: *The National Heart, Lung, and Blood Institute*

Counting the overweight bodies

Some people think the heat radiating from millions of well-padded Americans and Canadians may be causing global warming. If the trend continues, they suggest the whole darned planet may spontaneously combust. Poof!

A joke? Well, not entirely. According to the National Health and Nutrition Examination Survey (NHANES), as the following table shows, more than 60 percent of U.S. adults are either overweight or obese, a percentage 14 percent higher than in 1988 to 1994.

U.S. Adults	1976–1980	1988–1994	1999–2000
Overweight (BMI greater than or equal to 25.0)	27%	56%	64%
Obese (BMI greater than or equal to 30.0)	15%	23%	31%

The United States's neighbors to the north have nothing to brag about, either. According to Statistics Canada, by 1997 and 1998, a quarter of Canada's women and more than a third of men were overweight.

Canadian Population with BMI Greater than 27	1994–1995	1997–1998
Men	34%	37%
Women	22%	26%

These statistics are all the more reason to find a safe, effective way to lose the pounds that raise your risk of health problems, including heartburn and reflux.

Time in! To use the original BMI equation, Americans, who measure weight in pounds and height in inches, must convert these measurements to metric equivalents:

- ✔ To convert pounds to kilograms, divide the pounds by 2.2.
- ✔ To convert inches to meters, divide the inches by 39.

Or, heck, Yanks can simply use a BMI equation based on inches and pounds, with one extra step, multiplying the whole thing by 705:

$$BMI = W/H^2 \times 705$$

Once again, plug your personal numbers into the BMI equation. For example, if you're 5'4" tall, or 64 inches in America (1.626 meters in the metric version), and weigh 140 pounds (63.5 kilograms), the American BMI calculation looks like this:

$$BMI = W/H^2 \times 705 =$$

$$[140 \text{ pounds}/(64 \text{inches} \times 64 \text{inches})] \times 705 =$$

$$(140 \text{ pounds}/4,096 \text{ sq. inches}) \times 705 =$$

$$24.10 \text{ BMI}$$

Figuring out where your figures fit

After you check out the BMI chart, figure out where your figure fits in the following list. Based on information from the NIH, Health Canada, and the World Health Organization (WHO), the list shows how American, Canadian, and International BMI experts classify your body.

- ✔ **Underweight:** BMI lower than 18.5
- ✔ **Acceptable:** BMI between 18.5 and 24.9
- ✔ **Overweight:** BMI between 25.0 to 29.9
- ✔ **Obese:** BMI over 30

BMI is a neat tool, but as every fan of home improvement knows, even the very best tool doesn't work for every job — or in this case, every body. Check out the following areas where BMI doesn't necessarily apply:

- ✔ **Athletes:** BMI isn't always accurate for athletes. Muscle tissue is denser and heavier than fatty tissue; a lean athlete may weigh more but have a lower risk of weight-related health problems than a fluffy coach potato.

- ✔ **Children:** BMI isn't for kids. Chubby children's bodies are still growing and changing. Overweight toddlers and teens need a doctor's advice on weight loss.

- ✔ **Pregnant or nursing women:** BMI isn't a safe guide for women who are pregnant or nursing. The extra weight isn't useless fat: it's the Next Generation!

- ✔ **Senior citizens:** A number considered slightly puffy for a younger person may be protective after 65 when fat padding can soften the impact of an accidental fall on vulnerable hip bones.

Choosing a Healthful Weight Control Program

Wanna lose weight? Stop eating. Oops. Incomplete question. Wrong answer. How about wanna lose weight *and stay healthy?* You've got three practical options:

✔ A carb-based, controlled-fat diet

✔ A high-protein, low-carb diet

✔ Everything else

Wait, I see a hand in the back there. Oh, you want to know about low-calorie diets. Well, don't tell a soul, but virtually *every* weight-loss plan that actually works performs its magic by cutting calories. Notice I said "virtually," because as you read in the section "Adding up calories," later in this chapter, one serious study on one controversial diet has come up with one heck of a puzzling conclusion on whether calories count.

Counting calories

As my book *Nutrition For Dummies* (Wiley) explains, machines burn fuel, such as gasoline or kerosene, to get the energy (heat) they need to move. Living things — dogs, cats, ferrets, bacteria, you, and I — burn (metabolize) food to produce the energy (heat) to move around. Nutritionists measure the energy people get from food in units called *calories.*

Take in more calories than you use each day, and you gain weight. Take in fewer, and you lose weight. Isn't that amazing?

The magic number is 3,500 — the calorie equivalent of one pound of body fat. If you reduce your calorie consumption by 500 calories a day, even without becoming more active, you'll lose one pound in about seven days. If you go the other way and take in an extra 500 calories a day without doing any more work, seven days later, you'll weigh one pound more.

In order to control your weight, you need to know how many calories you require to maintain a healthful weight. Luckily, the National Academy of Sciences has done the math for you. The academy's newest recommendations, shown in Table 13-2, are based (for the first time ever) on actual measurements, the amount of daily calories burned by healthy people who maintain a normal body weight, defined as Body Mass Index (BMI) between 18.5 and 24.9. Note that the lower weight is BMI 18.5; the higher weight is BMI 24.9.

Like BMI, these new calorie recommendations are unisex, based on weight and height rather than gender. But the average man has proportionately more muscle than the average woman, so he can consume about 10 percent more calories per day without gaining weight. As a rule, therefore, a woman's calorie count should be at the lower end of the range; a man's, at the upper end. Hey, nobody ever said life was fair!

If you don't find your body on this chart — for example, you're a 6'5", 210-pound man and this chart only goes up to 6'3" — check with your doctor to determine the correct amount of calories you need to keep your energy high and your weight where it should be.

Table 13-2	Calories Required to Maintain a Healthful Weight
Height and Weight (Active Men and Women)	*Recommended Daily Calories*
5'1"/ 98 lbs	2,104–2,305
5'1"/124 lbs	2,290–2,615
5'3"/104 lbs	2,185–2,397
5'3"/141 lbs	2,383–2,727
5'5"/111 lbs	2,267–2,490
5'5"/150 lbs	2,477–2,842
5'7"/118 lbs	2,350–2,586
5'7"/159 lbs	2,573–2,959
5'9"/125 lbs	2,434–2,683
5'9"/169 lbs	2,670–3,078
5'11"/132 lbs	2,519–2,782
5'11"/178 lbs	2,769–3,200
6'1"/139 lbs	2,605–2,883
6'1"/188 lbs	2,869–3,325
6'3"/147 lbs	2,693–2,986
6'3"/199 lbs	2,971–3,452

Carbing down the pounds

This heading could also read "Curbing your calories with carbs" or "Carving the pounds with carbs," but they all mean the following:

Carbohydrate-based/controlled-fats diets such as the American Heart Association (AHA) Step I and Step II Diets, the American Diabetes Association Diet, and any diet based on the U.S. Departments of Agriculture and Health and Human Services (USDA/HHS) food guide pyramid emphasize low-fat foods such as grains, fruits, and veggies plus reduced-fat dairy products and controlled servings of high-protein foods such as meat, fish, and poultry.

The scientific name for this kind of diet is *carbohydrate-based/low cholesterol/controlled fat.* The first two phrases are self-explanatory, but why *controlled fat* rather than simply *low fat?* Because this diet tells you to choose fats that protect your heart (unsaturated fats) in place of fats that clog your arteries (saturated fats). Are you a bit shaky on the actual definition of saturated versus unsaturated? Check out *Nutrition For Dummies* (Wiley), which has a whole chapter devoted to distinguishing among good, bad, and totally horrible fats in food, including diagrams of the real molecules.

Benefits of a carb-based/controlled-fat diet

People who eat a carb-based/controlled-fat diet enjoy the following benefits:

- ✔ **This diet tastes good:** On this diet, you can eat virtually every food in the human pantry. The sole requirement is that you limit how much you eat. For example, even high-fat, high-cholesterol red meat is hunky-dory every once in a while as long as you limit your serving to 3 ounces, a portion about the size of a deck of cards.

- ✔ **This diet is really healthful:** The variety of food practically guarantees that you get all the vitamins and minerals you need from what you eat rather than from a supplement. As a bonus, emphasizing plant foods means you get lots of *phytochemicals* (*phyto* equals *plant*) reputed to reduce the risk of cancer and protect your vision among other benefits.

Variations on a carb-based/controlled-fat diet

The Pritikin Plan and the Ornish Diet, named after Nathan Pritikin and Dean Ornish, the men who invented them, are strict versions of the basic carb-based/controlled-fat meal plan. Pritikin allows only 15 percent of your calories from fat, while Ornish allows a measly 10 percent.

As a result, the food choices are so limited that even the AHA considers the Ornish Diet too restrictive for most people. On the other hand, if you're a Bad Heart Baby whose father had a heart attack before age 50 (mother, before age 60), or if you've had intimations of mortality yourself (very high cholesterol that doesn't respond to the moderate AHA diet), you may want to ask your doctor about Pritikin and Ornish. You don't want to plunge into these diets without a helping hand.

In the past ten years, food marketers have taken advantage of the popularity of carb-based/controlled-fats diets by promoting "fat-free" foods. However, fat-free-food manufacturers substitute flavor ingredients (read: sugar) for fat, which may convert a diet aid into a diet trap. Remember, calories do count. Whether you get calories from fat or from carbs, they add up to pounds.

Confusing carb terms

As you can see in Figure 13-1, the Nutrition Facts label shows the gram contents of carbohydrates, dietary fiber, and — sometimes — sugars.

Figure 13-1:
Carb copy.

Nutrition Facts
Serving size: 1/2 cup (114g)
Servings per container: 4

Amount per serving

Calories 90   Calories from fat 30

	% Daily Value*
Total Fat 3g	**5%**
Saturated Fat 0g	**0%**
Cholesterol 0mg	**0%**
Sodium 300mg	**13%**
Total Carbohydrate 13g	**4%**
Dietary Fiber 3g	**12%**
Sugars 3g	
Protein 3g	

Vitamin A 80%	•	**Vitamin C** 60%
Calcium 4%	•	**Iron** 4%

*Percent Daily Values are based on a 2,000 calorie diet. Your daily values may be higher or lower depending on your calorie needs:

		Calories	2,000	2,500
Total Fat	Less than		65g	80g
Sat Fat	Less than		20g	25g
Cholesterol	Less than		300mg	300mg
Sodium	Less than		2,400mg	2,400mg
Total Carbohydrate			300g	375g
Dietary Fiber			25g	30g

Calories per gram:
Fat 9 • Carbohydrate 4 • Protein 4

Now, *carbohydrates, sugars,* and *dietary fiber* are good, clear English words. But what in the world are *digestible carbs, nonimpact carbs,* and *effective carbs?* These are terms I found (a) in the Atkins Diet (more about that in the "Using protein to fight fat" section later in this chapter), and (b) on the labels for some carb-free meal replacement bars.

The terms *digestible carbs* and *effective carbs* refers to carbohydrates, such as sugar, that your body can digest. The term *nonimpact carbs* refers to carbohydrates such as dietary fiber and non-nutritive sweeteners such as saccharin, which your body doesn't digest and which therefore don't provide any nutrients, including calories. Although dietary fiber is included in a food's total carbohydrate count, it has no impact on your body's carb level, so you don't have to count it when you're counting carbs.

Using protein to fight fat

As you can see in Table 13-3, a high-protein/low-carb weight-loss plan, such as the Atkins Diet or the South Beach Diet, is the exact opposite of a carb-based/controlled-fat diet. But are the health effects of the high-protein/low-carb diet also the opposite?

Table 13-3	Carb-Based versus High Protein	
Characteristics	*Carb-Based*	*High Protein*
Food choices	Normal variety: Emphasizes plant foods	Restricted choices: Emphasizes foods from animals
Food servings	Measured portions	No limits for high protein foods; limits on carbohydrate foods
Total fat content	Low	High
Cholesterol content	Low	Moderate to high
Saturated fat content	Low	Moderate to high

Intuitively, your brain says, "Yes. Eating lots of fatty, high-protein foods makes me fat and sends my cholesterol sky-high. Not to mention my doctor is telling me that high-fat foods will loosen my LES and make my heartburn worse."

If I were writing these paragraphs a few years ago, I would have agreed with your brain. But guess what? Although conventional wisdom says the heavy dose of high-fat foods on a protein-based diet should make heartburn worse, the anecdotal evidence — what people who've tried the high-protein diet say — doesn't agree. Maybe the effect of lowering your weight carries more weight than the effect of high-fat foods on your heartburn symptoms. Stay tuned. Sooner or later someone or some study is sure to solve this mystery.

As for cholesterol, to the immense surprise of nutrition professionals everywhere in the galaxy, 2003 produced an explosion of new studies suggesting that high-protein/low-carb diets may actually take off unwanted pounds and lower your cholesterol.

✔ First, researchers from the Weight and Eating Disorders Program of the University of Pennsylvania School of Medicine, Washington University (St. Louis), and the University of Colorado divided a number of obese men and women weighing an average of 216 pounds into two groups. The first group got the Atkins Diet; the second, a carb-based/low-calorie diet. In the first three months, the Atkins dieters lost twice as much weight as the carb group. Ditto at six months. At the one-year mark, both groups had lost about the same amount of weight, but the Atkins dieters had significantly greater increases in good cholesterol (HDL) and their triglycerides, another risk factor for heart disease, were lower.

✔ Another group of Penn scientists at the Philadelphia VA Medical Center ran a six-month study with the same two diets. The results were similar: greater weight losses and reductions in triglycerides among people on the high-protein/low-carb regimen.

✔ Duke University researchers reported on a 120-person study in which volunteers were randomly assigned to either the high-protein Atkins Diet or the carb-based AHA diet. After six months, the Atkins people had lost an average of 31 pounds compared with 20 pounds for the carb-based dieters. Atkins dieters increased their HDLs (good cholesterol) and lowered their triglycerides.

How can this be, the nutrition establishment wondered? The obvious answer seems to be calories, because a high-protein diet is more satisfying and filling, so people end up eating less. Or maybe in a high-protein diet, the food choices are so boring that people don't eat as much.

So, a high-protein/low-carb weight-loss plan is the way to go, right? Not so fast.

Adding up calories

The Harvard study ran for 12 weeks and looked at 21 overweight volunteers in three groups:

✔ Group No.1 ate a carb-based/low-fat diet with 1,500 calories a day for women and 1,800 calories a day for men.

✔ Group No.2 ate a high-protein/low-carb diet with the same amount of calories.

✔ A luckier group No.3 ate the high-protein/low-carb diet with an extra 300 calories a day, which adds up to an extra 25,200 calories over 12 weeks. At 3,500 per pound of body fat, that should have added on an extra 7 pounds.

But guess what? The dieters in group No.3 lost just as much weight as those in group No.1. Pretty interesting, wouldn't you say?

The nutrition establishment was just as surprised about the results. As a result, these nutrition experts turned to physiological chemistry to explain the unexpected results.

Countering with chemistry

Your body runs on the energy supplied by *glucose* (sugar). Your primary source of glucose is carbohydrates. Pulling energy out of fats and protein is hard work that produces lots of waste in the form of water, which explains why people on a high-protein/low-carb diet run to the bathroom more often to relieve themselves.

The water loss also produces a fast, satisfying drop in weight, perhaps as much as seven pounds in four days. If you do drop seven pounds in four days as some high-protein/low-carb diets promise, you can reasonably assume that:

- ✔ A pound or two is fat.
- ✔ Five or six pounds are water, muscle tissue, water-soluble vitamins, and minerals (yes, that's why these diets recommend a supplement).

The fat pounds may stay off, but the water loss is strictly temporary. After you start eating carbs again, your body will happily revert to conserving water by pulling energy from sugars and starches. You seem to "gain back" weight, but you're simply re-establishing your normal fluid balance.

Can this explanation clarify why people lose weight on high-protein/low-carb diets even when they consume extra calories? Sorry, I don't have a clue. But neither does anyone else right now. Wait a few of years. A couple of confirming studies may answer that question. Science has a way of doing that.

Despite its benefits, a high-protein/low-carb diet may be so stingy with carbohydrates that it lacks sufficient amounts of important foods including milk and plants that contribute vital nutrients such as

- ✔ **Bone-building calcium:** Yes, you can have cheese, but ounce for ounce, cheese has less calcium than milk.
- ✔ **Heart-healthy folate:** When you start, Atkins permits three cups of salad and vegetables a day. This amount has less than half the recommended daily intake of folate, a B vitamin that not only protects your heart but also reduces the risk of birth defects.
- ✔ **Potassium:** Once again, the veggie allowance may not provide a sufficient amount of an important nutrient. Without enough potassium, you may feel dizzy; a serious potassium deficiency might even stop your heart.

To compensate for nutrients lost through a lack of carbohydrates, most protein-based diets recommend daily vitamin/mineral supplements, at least in the first, strict "induction" phase of the regimen. Don't ignore this serious advice. Discuss it with your doctor. Promise? Good. You're one smart cookie. Wait, no cookies, this is a low-carb diet. Sorry about that.

Simple versus complex

Some high-protein/low-carb programs such as the South Beach Diet make a big fuss about good carbs and bad carbs, by which they mean sugars (bad) and other carbs (good).

In fact, all carbohydrates are made of units (molecules) of sugar, but not all carbs are sweet because the word "sugar" in this instance refers to a specific chemical structure, not a flavor.

To explain that, I need to clarify a few points about carbohydrates. You can also check out my book *Nutrition For Dummies* (Wiley) for a more in-depth conversation.

✔ Fact No. 1: The word *carbohydrate* comes from *carbon* (carbo-) and *water* (hydr-).

✔ Fact No. 2: All carbs are made of units of sugar.

✔ Fact No. 3: Depending on how many sugar units a carbohydrate has or how the units are attached to one another, a carbohydrate is either *simple* or *complex*.

A *simple carbohydrate* has only one or two units of sugar. A carb with one sugar unit is a *monosaccharide* (*mono* = one; *saccharide* = sugar). Examples of monosaccharides are *fructose*

("fruit sugar") and *glucose* ("blood sugar" — the sugar produced when you digest carbs).

A carb with two sugar units is a *disaccharide* (*di* = two). The most familiar disaccharide is *sucrose* ("table sugar"), one unit of fructose plus one unit of glucose.

Complex carbohydrates, sometimes labeled *polysaccharides* (*poly* = many), have more than two units of sugar. *Raffinose,* a complex carb in potatoes, beans, and beets, has one unit each of galactose, glucose, and fructose. *Stachyose,* a complex carb in veggies, has one fructose unit, one glucose unit, and two galactose units. *Starch,* a complex carbohydrate in potatoes, pasta, and rice, has many units of glucose.

Dietary fiber, a special kind of carb, is a polysaccharide. But the human gut lacks the enzymes required to separate its sugar units, so eating dietary fiber doesn't give you any energy (calories) or nutrients.

Your body digests simple carbs faster than complex ones, so you get a faster energy rush from, says, sucrose, than you do from starch. In the end, though, all carbs become glucose, which means all carbs are good sources of energy.

Examining all those other weight-loss diets

After you take a serious look at carb-based weight-loss diets and protein-based ones, a funny thought may come creeping into your mind. You may wonder: Aren't all these diets either a variation on one of these themes or a tad weird? What do I mean by weird? I mean

✔ A diet that concentrates on one food or group of foods, such as grapefruit, celery, fruit, or veggies. The "magic" food or food group supposedly has super-special powers to burn fat or rev up your metabolism. The result is a very low-calorie, nutrient-deficient regimen so boring that nobody can stand it for more than a week.

✔ A diet that offers strange meal plans like not eating fruit with meat because "your body can't handle two kinds of food at one time." (Your body uses different enzymes to digest the carbohydrates in fruits and the proteins and fats in meat, and you're perfectly capable of chewing gum and walking . . . no, I mean secreting both kinds of enzymes at the same time.)

✔ A diet that relies on special secret products sold only by the guru who made up the diet. Guess who profits here? (Not you or me!) I say it again; you're a smart cookie.

Making a sensible weight-control choice

Carbohydrates versus proteins. Proteins versus carbohydrates. Which way wins? Perhaps the best choice is a reasonable compromise between the two contenders.

The high-protein/low-carb diet is great at dropping pounds fast, which makes you feel that *this time* you really will lose the weight that's bugging you. But the lack of food choices gets boring after a while, and you may begin to feel that if you don't eat some carbs, even a piece of plain dry toast, you'll die. I understand. I've been there.

The carb-based/controlled-fat diet takes a bit longer to prove its worth, but it's an excellent maintenance regimen that allows you at least small portions of every food on the planet. You can live with it. Trust me. I've been there, too.

R.I.P. Robert Atkins

In the 30 years after publishing the first edition of *Dr. Atkins' Diet Revolution,* Robert C. Atkins was a continuing presence on the international bestsellers' lists. One book alone — *Dr. Atkins' New Diet Revolution* (Avonbooks, 1992) — sold more than 10 million copies in 10 years to secure a place as one of the top-50 bestselling books of all time.

But bestseller or not, Atkins couldn't get any respect from his peers who criticized his theory that eating high-fat foods could take off pounds and improve health.

Not until after until after his death in April 2003 following an accidental fall did the evidence begin to appear suggesting that he may have had a point after all. However, today the controversy continues.

The 30/30 dream

Can you lose 30 pounds in 30 days? No way say the guys and gals at the American Society of Bariatric Physicians, a group of doctors specializing in weight control who point out that to lose one pound of body fat, you must cut your calorie intake by 3,500 calories. To lose 30 pounds in 30 days, you need to cut back 105,000 calories ($30 \times 3,500$ calories = 105,000 calories). A person consuming 2,800 calories a day (more than most American women eat each day) takes in a mere 84,000 calories in 30 days. If this person were to stop eating entirely for 30 days, she would still have to get rid of another 21,000 calories to reach 105,000.

So how about starting with proteins (plus the requisite supplement), and then switching — gradually — to carbs. (A gradual switch is important because it prevents an instantaneous bounce-back as your body adjusts to the added carbs.) As the ancient Greeks used to say, "Everything in moderation."

Working Off Your Reflux

Ordinarily, exercise is good for you. Moving your body strengthens your muscles and bones, revs up your brain, sharpens your immune system, and generally improves your mood. To save time and space, I put all this good stuff into Table 13-4, which shows exactly how a regular exercise program tunes up your various parts.

Table 13-4	Tuning Up and Turning On
Body Part	*What Exercise Does*
Blood (fats)	Lowers total cholesterol. Lowers levels of low-density lipoproteins (LDLs; "bad" cholesterol). Raises levels of high-density lipoproteins (HDLs; "good" cholesterol). Lowers levels of triglycerides.
Blood vessels	Increases blood flow. Relaxes blood vessels. Reduces risk of high blood pressure. Reduces risk of stroke.
Bones	Reduces natural loss of bone tissue. Lowers risk of osteoporosis.

(continued)

Table 13-4 *(continued)*

Body Part	What Exercise Does
Brain	Increases flow of oxygenated blood to brain tissue. Improves brain function. Increases production of *endorphins,* natural calming compounds that improve mood and alleviate pain. Improves sleeps.
Digestive tract	Quickens movement of food through intestinal tract. Reduces risk of constipation.
Fatty tissue	Reduces amount.
Immune system	Improves immune response.
Lungs	Improves elasticity of lung tissue. Increases respiration.
Muscles	Strengthens and enlarges muscle tissue.
Miscellaneous	Quickens metabolism. Promotes weight loss. Raises body temperature.

Look close. What's missing from this list? Aha! You got it! Exercise does have benefits for your digestive tract, but preventing reflux isn't one of them. In fact, working out may have exactly the opposite effect.

According to www.heartburnhelp.com, one of the useful Web sites in Chapter 21, the following studies indicate that as many as one in every seven heartburn sufferers may experience exercise-related reflux:

✔ In an Oklahoma Foundation for Digestive Research survey of 319 athletes, 43 percent developed heartburnlike symptoms while working out, and the researchers found that more-intense workouts produced more-intense symptoms.

✔ Two additional studies — one with cyclists, the other with weightlifters — produced similar results. Nine out of ten cyclists developed mild reflux. Ditto for weightlifters.

But what exactly are the links between exercise and reflux?

✔ **Physical activity:** Being active slows the exit of food from your stomach, leaving plenty of food sloshing about and ready to back up into your esophagus as you move around.

> ✔ **Tense muscles:** Tensing your abdominal muscles (in this case to lift weights) pushes your stomach up against your LES and loosening it — the main cause of heartburn and reflux! Simple aerobics can produce the same distress.

> ✔ **Bent bodies:** Bending at the waist (like over the handlebars of a bike) shortens the distance between your stomach and your esophagus, producing pretty much the same results as those linked to tense muscles.

Your task is to find an exercise regimen and a meal schedule that doesn't exacerbate your reflux. What? You were expecting me to say you need to forego exercise entirely? Given all that good stuff in Table 13-4, not a chance!

Eating smart for a comfortable workout

If working out wakes up your heartburn, and even the thought of exercise makes you want to run away and hide in an antacid bottle, the National Heartburn Alliance (NHBA) has some advice for you.

Visit the alliance's Web site (www.heartburnalliance.com) for expert advice, or you can skim through my *For Dummies*–friendly version right here. If you choose the latter, do check out the Web site, which is a treasure trove of heartburn help.

Avoiding food right before exercising

Your mother probably told you to wait an hour after eating before diving into the pool. As an adult with heartburn, waiting two hours after eating before you exercise is even safer. The one exception seems to be a leisurely after-meal walk. Yes, you're moving, but you're upright, which is one stratagem for avoiding heartburn.

Eating low-fat meals — in small portions

Think *low-fat* when planning pre-exercise meals.

> ✔ High-fat foods linger longer in your stomach, sort of like guests who don't take a hint to leave. The longer the high-fat foods linger, the higher the risk that they'll slip back through the LES to set off heartburn.

> ✔ Low-fat carbs are better behaved. They never overstay their welcome. Instead they exit your stomach fairly quickly, a digestive pattern that forms the basis for the old joke about being hungry an hour after eating Chinese food like chow mein — high-carb, low-fat veggie dishes. Now you know the joke isn't a joke; it's a digestive fact.

And keep the portions small. The reason for this piece of advice is self-evident. Small portions clear out of the stomach faster, providing the same benefits as low-fat foods.

Passing up personal heartburn triggers

In Chapter 6, I list many common offenders that trigger heartburn, including citrus juices, chocolate candy, mint flavorings, caffeine, and bubbly beverages (think soda pop or even sparkling water).

But remember: Each of us is an individual. You may react to one food that doesn't ring even the smallest bell in my digestive tract. And vice versa, too. This list, therefore, is open to personal additions and subtractions. Be sure to subtract from your diet the ones that add up to heartburn for you.

Drinking plenty of water (maybe even in your sports drink)

Water is an essential ingredient of every successful exercise program. Not only does drinking enough water replenish the liquids lost when you perspire, but it also helps move food down through the digestive tract, away from the vulnerable LES. Furthermore, adding water to your sports drink dilutes the high concentration of carbohydrates in the liquid so your stomach empties faster after you take a swig. ***Don't forget:*** The less food and liquids sloshing around in your stomach, the lower your risk of bounce-back reflux.

Having an antacid for dessert

If you aren't regularly taking a 24-hour-pill, such as an H2 blocker or a proton pump inhibitor (PPI), you may find that grabbing an over-the-counter (OTC) antacid before you exercise goes a long way toward reducing the incidence and severity of your exercise-related heartburn. Ditto for taking an antacid if heartburn begins during (or after) exercise.

Check with your doctor before adding any new meds. And, naturally, if you're not sure what an H2 blocker or a PPI is, you can check it out in Chapter 10. More smart-cookie behavior.

Adapting your exercise to your heartburn

Define the word *exercise.* No, this isn't a trick. Many people think the word *exercise* means professional-level sports, a 10-mile run, or a hop-'til-you-drop celebrity workout. These people are wrong.

Exercise is just plain movement. You don't have to be training for the Olympics; your favorite sport — golf, tennis, or even Ping-Pong — is good exercise. Cleaning house is good exercise, especially if, as the AHA suggests, "you vacuum vigorously." Maybe to music?

Walking is also good exercise. No, walking is *great* exercise, especially for people with reflux. Unlike jogging, which bounces your insides about, walking is a smooth interplay of muscles that moves virtually every part of your body (swing those arms! shift those eyes! turn that head!).

Best of all, walking is terrific for people with heartburn because it avoids bending your body or tensing your muscles, the maneuvers that so often set off reflux (see Figure 13-2)

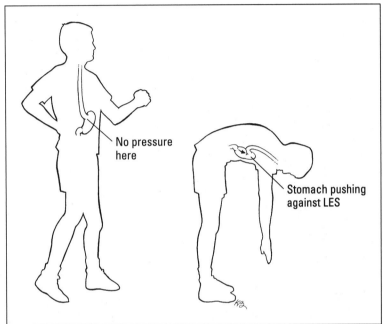

Figure 13-2:
Keeping
your
exercise
straight.

And Figure 13-3 shows precisely how simple changes can make some forms of exercise kinder to your digestive tract.

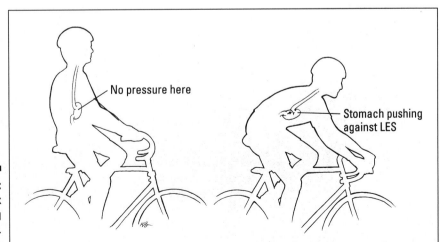

Figure 13-3:
Reflux
biking
basics.

Recognizing when exercise may not bother your reflux

Some people with heartburn never have a problem when they exercise. I say, good for them, the lucky souls! For example, if your doctor is treating your reflux with a 24-hour medication, you may have absolutely no problem with any exercise program. Hop, skip, jump, jog, do whatever — the new heart-burn meds may be so effective that you can position yourself in any position without setting off fire alarms in your esophagus. Ain't medical science grand?

Setting sensible exercise standards

Pretend you've never heard the words *heartburn* and *reflux*. But you've definitely heard of exercise, and you've decided you want to try some in order to

- ✔ Trim some pounds
- ✔ Harden some muscles
- ✔ Improve your circulation
- ✔ Generally feel better

How do you proceed? Well, don't just do something. Sit there! Yes, you heard me right. Exercising safely and effectively isn't a matter of jumping into the pool and hoping you'll float. The better way is to consider the options, lay out some ground rules, put on your water wings — and then jump. For example:

Being reasonable

You're not planning to turn pro; you just want to feel better, which may include accommodating your exercise to your heartburn. So stick to simple stuff like walking rather than jogging, or stretching for yoga or pilates (read all about it in *Yoga For Dummies* by Georg Feuerstein and Larry Payne or *Pilates For Dummies* by Ellie Herman Wiley) rather than bouncing about on parallel bars. Doing that isn't a surrender. It's an intelligent plan.

Picking a play you enjoy

Yes, I say *play!* The AHA calls *play* "activities that are fun, not exhausting." If you hate football, loathe jogging, despise aerobics, and can't stand to get your hair wet in a pool, an exercise regimen that includes these activities won't last out the weekend in your life. So what good do they do you in the long run? None. Pick something you enjoy doing.

Setting a schedule and sticking to it

To be valuable, your exercise should be consistent. Better an hour's walk every day than a "beat-'em-up, burn-'em-down" marathon once a year. And believe it or not, you don't have to do your hour all at once. You can break it down into three 20-minute power walks and still get all the benefits.

Keeping your standards high

If you decide to join a fitness program or a gym, look for serious credentials. The American College of Sports Medicine (ACSM), the National Academy of Sports Medicine (NASM), the American Council on Exercise (ACE), and the National Strength and Conditioning Association (NSCA) all provide certification tests for fitness professionals. So check out the framed diplomas on your instructor's wall? No diplomas? No dice.

Checking with your doctor

Don't start your new regimen without asking your doctor if you're fit for the program you've chosen.

Relying on the best

Read more about how to create a sensible exercise program in *Fitness For Dummies* by Suzanne Schlosberg and Liz Neporent (Wiley). Go and get your own copy. Like, now. Unless, of course, you're first raring to read more about heartburn and reflux, which, if that's the case, flip to the table of contents for the next subject you want to uncover.

Chapter 14

Healing Heartburn with Healthy Habits

*T*his short chapter contain stuff you may have seen or heard a hundred times. But you can't write a book about reflux without mentioning that you can ease your heartburn by (a) giving up tobacco, (b) using alcohol in moderation (or not at all), and (c) getting a good night's sleep.

So, humor me. Even if you've already learned your (a)(b)(c)'s, take some time to flip through these pages. Who knows? You may pick up something interesting. Like the year smoking was banned on domestic flights in the United States. Or who wrote "Tobacco is a filthy weed . . . ." In other words, don't skip this chapter too quickly!

Snuffing Out Heartburn

Vietnam-era protesters once chanted, "War is not healthy for children and other living things." Well, smoking isn't healthy for children and other living things, either.

Experts estimate that tobacco smoke contains as many as 4,000 different chemicals, including *carcinogens* (substances that cause cancer). The three main components of tobacco smoke, however, are tar, nicotine, and carbon monoxide — nasty players all:

- ✔ **Tar:** This sticky mixture of tobacco-smoke compounds includes poisons and carcinogens that irritate your mouth and esophagus, stick to your lungs, and kill or incapacitate the tiny hairs called *cilia* that ordinarily sweep debris from your lungs to keep them clean. The result is (you got it) a cough.

- ✔ **Nicotine:** This chemical delivers the "hit" you get when you inhale tobacco smoke. Nicotine is an addictive drug that revs up your nervous system, speeds up your heart, and raises your blood pressure by constricting small blood vessels under the skin. Nicotine also raises your risk of heart attack by making *platelets* (small particles in your blood) more likely to stick together and form an artery-blocking blood clot. These physical reactions result in a higher risk of heart attack.

- ✔ **Carbon monoxide:** This gas can displace the oxygen normally carried by red blood cells to every tissue in your body, slowly suffocating cells and organs. As a result, you may gasp for every little breath you take.

Every time you suck on a lit stick of tobacco — ugh! burning dead leaves! — tar, nicotine, carbon monoxide, and the other ingredients in that blue tobacco smoke

- ✔ Give you bad breath

- ✔ Irritate your gums and loosen your teeth

- ✔ Wrinkle your face

- ✔ Weaken your bones

- ✔ Speed up your heartbeat

- ✔ Narrow your arteries

- ✔ Increase your risk of lung cancer, bladder cancer, kidney cancer, esophageal cancer, and cancer of the pancreas

Wait! Something's missing! Right: I haven't mentioned that smoking also raises your risk of reflux and heartburn.

Linking tobacco to heartburn

Honesty compels me to admit that not every study on smoking and heartburn shows a link between the two. But most experts agree the link exists. Indeed, the National Heartburn Alliance (NHBA) — you can read more about it in Chapter 21 — notes that at least one large study shows that smoking

- ✔ Increases esophageal exposure to stomach acid more than 50 percent.

- ✔ Increases incidents of daytime reflux 114 percent (during the day, when you're standing up, gravity normally keep stomach acid in the stomach).

Christening tobacco

People have been calling tobacco nasty names ("coffin nails" for cigarettes comes quickly to mind) ever since European explorers first brought the fragrant leaves back from the New World to the Old World. But if you want to touch off a true literary-criticism debate, try asking who wrote this little ditty:

Tobacco is a filthy weed,
That from the devil doth proceed;
That drains your purse, that burns your clothes,
That makes a chimney of your nose.

Some experts vote for that old favorite, Anonymous, who is often credited with penning the poem around the middle of the 17th century. Other sources — such as the prestigious *Bartlett's Familiar Quotations* (Justin Kaplan, editor; Little, Brown & Company) — point to Boston physician Benjamin Waterhouse, one of the first three professors at the new Harvard School of Medicine in 1792 and the doctor who vaccinated Oliver Wendell Holmes, another Boston physician and author.

These unpleasant effects are almost certainly due to the fact that inhaling tobacco smoke loosens the lower esophageal sphincter (LES), the "trapdoor" between your esophagus and stomach, which is supposed to close tight after you swallow so that the acid contents of your stomach don't *reflux* (flow back into your esophagus). Want to know more about the LES? Look no further than Chapter 2.

But the bad news doesn't stop there. Smoking not only makes the LES wobbly. Dragging that smoke into your lungs also worsens the reflux-related injury to the delicate lining of your esophagus because tobacco smoke

- ✔ Irritates your esophagus.

- ✔ Decreases the secretion of saliva, a fluid that otherwise helps counter the acidity of any acidic stomach contents that flow back into the esophagus during reflux. As a result, it takes longer than normal to wash reflux material out of your esophagus.

- ✔ Changes the composition of saliva, which is normally *basic* (the opposite of acid). (See Chapter 2 for more on pH and basic versus acid.) As a result, saliva is less effective at neutralizing stomach juices that have crept into your esophagus.

- ✔ Reduces the healing powers of antireflux medicines (for more on medication options, check out Chapter 10).

When you come right down to it, smoking may be the only vice with absolutely, totally no redeeming virtue. But as an ex-smoker myself, I know how difficult quitting can be.

Leaving a losing habit

If you have heartburn and you smoke, quitting the latter can help make the former better. When you do decide to quit, and now is an excellent time, you have four clear options:

- ✔ You can just quit.
- ✔ You can quit with the help of medication.
- ✔ You can quit with the help of a behavior-modification program.
- ✔ You can try one from Column A, one from Column B, one from Column C — in other words, a sort of buffet approach to the matter at hand.

Deciding to stop smoking is truly a "whatever works" situation. Each of the four strategies listed above has good points and bad points. For a totally complete look at each and every point, you can pick up a copy of *Quitting Smoking For Dummies* by David Brizer, MD (Wiley), just about the best, most detailed guide you can get. But you came here for answers, so I'm going to give 'em to you.

Quitting cold turkey

Just stop. But give yourself an out. An about-to-be-ex-smoker's worst nightmare is waking up at 4 a.m. without a ciggie in the house. At that point, resolve dissolves in the frantic search through every drawer and coat pocket, and a not-so-stalwart sort-of-ex-smoker may succumb to a panic, rushing to the corner newsstand to buy a brand new pack of cigarettes. To keep your panic in check, keep a pack of cigarettes handy. Yes, you read that right: Keep the smokes available, but don't light up. Easier said than done? Sure.

Kicking the habit is easier if you do it in steps — one hour at a time, then one morning at a time, then one day at a time, and then one lifetime at a time. I don't know if any study supports this approach, but I used it when I stopped smoking, and it worked for me. Perhaps it can work for you, as well.

Easing anxiety

For some people, the path to a smoke-free Nirvana runs through a prescription for the antidepressant medication bupropion (Zyban).

In several well-controlled studies, Zyban alone — without counseling or any other therapy — enabled up to 50 percent of the people who took it to stay smoke-free for seven weeks and up to 23 percent to avoid cigarettes for at least a year. Those numbers may not sound all that impressive, but guess what? Only 4 to 7 percent of smokers who try to quit on their own make it for one full year without cigarettes. As a result, the Food and Drug Administration (FDA) has approved Zyban as a stop-smoking aid, and many insurance plans now pick up at least part of the cost.

Zyban does have some potential adverse effects — upset stomach, headache, insomnia, irritability in anyone who takes the drug, and seizures in people with a history of seizure disorders.

But Zyban therapy also has an interesting benefit in addition to its ability to help quell the craving for a smoke. Smokers who quit often gain weight. Zyban produces a slight weight loss. No smoking, the possibility of no weight gain, and insurance coverage? Gloriosky!

Replacing nicotine

In a world with a pill for every ill, I doubt anyone's surprised to hear that there are pills — and patches, nasal sprays, and chewing gums — that fight nicotine craving by delivering nicotine to your bloodstream without your having to inhale smoke.

These products — known collectively as *nicotine replacement therapy* (NRT) — deliver small doses of nicotine to your bloodstream without your having to inhale tobacco smoke with all its nasty gases and tars. Most cigarettes sold in the United States contain 10 mg (or more) of nicotine and deliver about 1 to 2 mg per smoked cigarette. The nicotine replacement products vary in nicotine dosage, but all are designed to reduce your craving for cigarettes by lessening common withdrawal symptoms, such as irritability, headache, sleep disturbances, and fatigue.

Table 14-1 lists the different kinds of NRT products available in the United States and Canada. NRT products are — yes, you got it — medicines. If you decide to try one, be sure to check with your doctor first.

Table 14-1	American and Canadian NRT			
Product Type	*Brand Names*	*Doses*	*Available in U.S.*	*Available in Canada*
Gum	Nicorette	2 mg	Y	Y
		4 mg	N	Y
	Nicorette DS	4 mg	Y	Y

(continued)

Table 14-1 *(continued)*

Product Type	Brand Names	Doses	Available in U.S.	Available in Canada
Patch	Nicoderm CQ and Nicotrol			
	16-hour	5,10,15 mg	Y	N
	24-hour	7 mg	Y	Y
		11 mg	Y	Y
		14 mg	Y	Y
		21 mg	Y	Y
		22 mg	Y	N
Nasal spray	Nicotrol	*	Y	Y
Inhaler	Nicotrol	**	Y	Y

*0.5 mg per spray; one spray in each nostril; maximum 5 doses per hour; by prescription only.
** Inhaler delivers 4 mg per dose; only 2 mg absorbed, by prescription only.
Sources: *Rybacki, J.J., Long, J.W., The Essential Guide to Prescription Drugs 2000 (New York, N.Y: Harper Perennial, 2000); The Physicians' Desk Reference 2001 (Montvale, NJ: Medical Economics Company, 2001)*

Modifying your behavior

Behavior modification aims to teach you how to avoid or ignore emotional and physical triggers, such as anxiety or nicotine craving, that tell you to light up. People learn in different ways. Some do better in a class; others respond to a book. Whichever works for you is your best solution.

For information about stop-smoking programs in your area, click on a reliable Web site, like the American Lung Association at www.lungusa.org or the Canadian Lung Association at www.lung.ca. You can find what you're looking for at both sites. Or you can call your local hospital or YMCA, which almost certainly has a stop-smoking program on premise.

Writing a word to the willing

Ending your relationship with tobacco isn't a Sunday walk in the park. Nicotine is such a rewarding drug that leaving it behind takes time and effort. Sometimes, it takes a lot of time and even more effort. Often, people who don't make it right away feel guilty. As they say in New Yawk — fuggeddaboudit!

Blowing smoke — away!

The idea that smoking is hazardous to your health is nothing new. For more than 100 years, American doctors and legislators have been trying to convince smokers to give up their cigarettes, cigars, and pipes. This list is a short guide to important stop-smoking moments.

1892 U.S. Senate's Committee on Epidemic Disease names cigarettes a public health hazard.

1917 At least 14 states have banned the possession, sale, manufacture, or use of cigarettes.

1929 U.S. Surgeon General says smoking makes women nervous insomniacs.

1959 American Cancer Society publishes figures showing male death rates are three times higher among smokers than among nonsmokers; five times higher for heavy smokers

1961 American Cancer Society, American Heart Association, American Public Health Association, and the National Tuberculosis Association ask President John F. Kennedy to create a panel to study the health effects of smoking.

1962 Surgeon General's Report names smoking a major health risk, linking it to rising cancer rates.

1963 U.S. government requires warning labels on cigarette packages.

1973 First nonsmoking sections are established for passengers on commercial airlines in United States.

1973 Arizona becomes the first state in the United States to regulate smoking.

1984 Comprehensive Smoking Education Act introduces rotating warnings for cigarette packs.

1987 U.S. Department of Health and Human Services bans smoking in its offices.

1990 Smoking banned on all U.S. domestic flights shorter than six hours.

1993 U.S. Environmental Protection Agency links secondhand smoke to health problems.

1994 Mississippi sues the tobacco industry for the cost of smoking-related health problems.

1995 California bans smoking in all indoor business and restaurants.

1997 Tobacco industry and state attorneys general agreement establishes ad restrictions, health warnings, funding for antismoking program, and healthcare payments to states.

1998 California bans smoking in bars and clubs.

1999 192 countries of the United Nations meet to draw up an antismoking treaty.

2003 New York (yes, New York) bans indoor smoking in all restaurants and bars throughout the state. So does the entire country of Ireland. If they can do it, so can you!

Not quitting forever the first time you quit smoking is neither a crime nor a moral failure. Neither is not making it the first 10 or 20 times. Every time you stop smoking, you keep your body free of tobacco-smoke glop for hours or days or weeks. Consider that an accomplishment to celebrate because, in the end, the only important thing is the end — of smoking.

Toasting the Pain-Free Life

Alcoholic beverages are among mankind's oldest home remedies and simple pleasures, so highly regarded that the ancient Greeks and Romans called wine a gift from the gods. As for distilled spirits, the Gaels (early inhabitants of Ireland) called them *uisgebeatha* (whis-*key*-ba). The French said *eau de vie* (o-duh-*vee*). The Scandinavians, *aquavit* (ah-*kwa*-veet). In any language, that means "water of life."

In my book *Nutrition For Dummies* (Wiley), I wrote an entire chapter on how alcohol affects your body. I cut to the chase here to explain precisely how alcoholic beverages may harm your digestive tract and — you knew this was coming, right? — raise your risk of reflux.

Explaining why alcohol raises your risk of reflux

Alcohol is an annoying irritant that affects virtually every part of your digestive tract. For example, alcohol

- Coagulates proteins on your tongue and the mucous membrane lining of your mouth, creating that slight burning sensation when you take a sip.
- Irritates and reddens the lining of your esophagus.
- Relaxes the muscles that should hold your LES shut.
- Makes your stomach step up its production of stomach acid and *histamine,* the same immune-system chemical that makes the skin around a mosquito bite red and itchy. (After you drink enough, you start to feel slightly queasy. Who wouldn't, with a stomach that looks like one big bug bite?)

And if that weren't enough, alcohol worsens any existing damage to your mouth and esophagus. Data from the American Cancer Society's Cancer Prevention 1 study show that people who take more than two drinks a day have a higher incidence of oral and esophageal cancer. Combining alcohol with tobacco is even more dangerous. In tandem, the pair can raise your risk of esophageal cancer *exponentially* (a scientific term used to describe enormous jumps in numbers).

How enormous? Well, if I say something doubles your risk, that means it increases your risk by 100 percent. Smoking plus drinking increases the risk of esophageal cancer by more than 150 times. For simplicity's sake, call it 160 times. When you set up these statements as mathematical equations, the numbers look like this:

- **Equation No. 1:** 2×2 (2×2 once) = 100 percent (double the risk)

- **Equation No. 2:** 2×2 (2×2 160 times) = 16,000 percent (160 times the risk)

Wow! That's exponential, all right. In fact, it may be a tad over the edge, statistics-wise. The main thing is that smoking + drinking = a higher risk to your esophagus than either smoking or drinking alone. Got it? Good!

Defining a drink

For most people with heartburn, one drink is safer than two drinks, and no drink is safest of all. But bodies differ, so your doctor — and your own digestive tract — are your best guides to your personal use of alcoholic drinks.

Which brings us to the perennial question, What's a drink, anyway? Table 14-2 has the answers. But, you say, the table has two different definitions. Yes, you get a choice. After all, as we all know, choices are the spice of life.

Table 14-2	What's One Drink?		
Source	*Beer*	*Wine*	*Spirits*
American Heart Association	12.0 oz.	4.0 oz.	1.0 oz. (100 proof) 1.5 oz. (80 proof)
Dietary Guidelines for Americans 2000	12.0 oz.	5.0 oz.	1.5 oz. (80 proof)

Grooving on grapes

Medical experts agree that alcoholic beverages lower your risk of heart disease. Some studies say that the beneficial ingredient is the alcohol itself. Many more, however, point to *resveratrol,* a naturally occurring compound in grape skin, pulp, and seeds (the parts of the fruit more widely used in red wines). Resveratrol is a *flavonoid,* an antioxidant that powers up other antioxidants, such as vitamin E and vitamin C, which prevent molecule fragments from linking up to form rogue molecules that damage body cells.

Juice from purple grapes has more resveratrol than the juice from red grapes, which has more resveratrol than the juice from white grapes (get the red wine connection?). To be even more specific, in 1998, a team of food scientists from the USDA Agricultural Research Service identified a native American grape, the muscadine, as an unusually potent source of resveratrol.

You can enjoy the benefits of resveratrol without risking the heartburn/reflux effects of alcohol.

Just eat grapes. Or better yet, drink grape juice. Ounce for ounce, you get more resveratrol from grape juice than from plain grapes and — as you can see in the following table — as much resveratrol as you get from wine. And, oh, yes — the darker the juice, the higher the resveratrol. In other words, three cheers for Concord grape juice!

Nutrient	Grape Juice (4 oz.)	Red Wine (4 oz.)
Water (oz.)	3.5	3.5
Calories	77	85
Carbohydrates (g)	19	2
Resveratrol (msg)*	320-640	320-640

*Mcg = Microgram = 1/1000th mg (milligram).
Source: USDA

This warning has nothing to do with reflux, but read it anyway. Some people are sensitive to or allergic to sulfites, compounds used as preservatives in some foods such as dried fruits and some wines. Exposure to sulfites can cause potentially serious allergic reactions for sensitive folks. To avoid problems, the government requires all alcohol products containing sulfites to say so on the label.

Getting a Good Night's Sleep

Nearly 80 percent of American adults with heartburn have nighttime reflux, a condition that the NHBA says

- ✔ Is more painful than daytime heartburn
- ✔ Deprives you of sleep

✔ Interferes with work the next day

✔ Interferes with your social life

✔ Causes more psychological distress than other chronic problems, such as hypertension and diabetes, and about as much stress as angina and congestive heart failure

Worse yet, much evidence suggests that nighttime reflux may be more damaging than daytime reflux because when you're lying down, the acid lingers longer in your esophagus. How damaging is "more" damaging? The American Gastroenterological Association (AGA) says *very.*

AGA is one of the oldest medical societies in the United States, so when these guys talk, everybody listens. In 2001, the AGA was talking about a Gallup nationwide telephone survey of 1,000 adults with at least one heartburn episode a week. The study data showed that people with *nocturnal* (a fancy word for nighttime) heartburn symptoms were 11 times more likely to develop esophageal cancer than those who don't, presumably because acid remains in the esophagus for longer periods of time while sufferers lie in bed.

As a result of the 2001 study, the AGA created the Nighttime Heartburn Relief Effort, an educational campaign for doctors and reflux patients. To find out more, go to the AGA Web site, www.gastro.org, and type "heartburn" into the search box on the homepage. This brings up several pages detailing studies, surveys, press releases, and self-help info on nighttime heartburn. To lessen your risk of nighttime reflux, read on.

Picking a comfy position

How you position your body when you settle down to sleep may affect your risk of developing heartburn during the night. Your goal is to keep your stomach on a lower level than your esophagus to minimize the possibility of stomach liquids flowing backwards to irritate the esophagus. Now, you know about interactive Web sites, right? Well, this section is interactive, too. Your cooperation is definitely required, step by step:

1. **Bookmark this page, turn back to Chapter 2, and check out the diagram of your *digestive tract,* which is essentially a long tube that starts at your mouth and ends at, well, the end.**

   Your stomach — a balloonlike organ behind your left ribs — is one part of the tube. Fix the pix firmly in your mind.

2. **Take this book into your bedroom. Lie down on your bed, flat on your back.**

   As Figure 14-1 shows — no, don't get up, just hold the book up so you can see the picture — when you lie flat, your digestive tract flattens out, too. As a result, acidic stomach liquids may flow easily back through a loose LES into your esophagus.

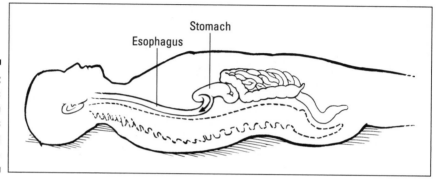

Figure 14-1: Acidic stomach contents sliding backwards.

3. **Lie on your right side. Hold this book up and stare at Figure 14-2.**

   See? When you lie on your right side, your stomach is higher than your esophagus, so those nasty stomach liquids can spill downhill into your esophagus. After the liquids have slid, the Law of Gravity says they ain't gonna flow back uphill into your stomach.

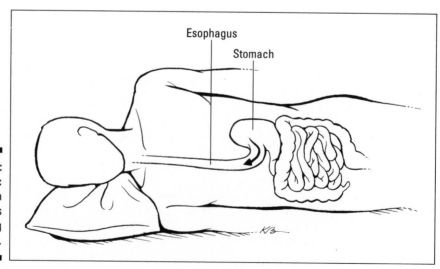

Figure 14-2: Acidic stomach contents rolling along.

4. Lie on your left side. Now focus on Figure 14-3.

This picture shows that when you lie on your left side, your stomach is lower than your esophagus, which means that the Law of Gravity is on your side, preventing those gastric liquids from flowing on what is now an uphill slope into your esophagus. Yeah!

Figure 14-3:
Lying on your left side helps prevent acidic stomach contents from entering the esoph-agus — happy bedtime.

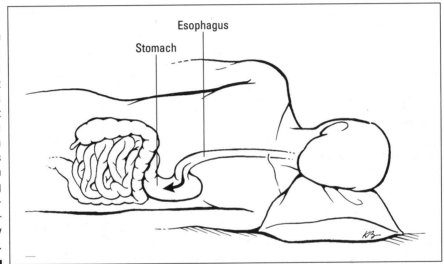

Esophagus

Stomach

5. Give yourself an extra lift. Slip a wedge-shaped pillow under your head (or under your mattress) to raise the head of the bed and keep your digestive tube on a downhill slope.

No guarantees, but like sleeping on your left side, sleeping on a wedge pillow may help ease nighttime reflux. For more info on fighting heart-burn with fashion and furniture (including more information on making the bed for a good night's sleep), see Chapter 16.

Altering your eating habits

REMEMBER

Are you the kind of person who crawls into bed with a book, some cookies, and a glass of milk? Not a good way to go. From now on, you can keep the book, but lose the milk and cookies. In fact, forget about food — any food — for at least two or three hours before you go to bed because a more-or-less empty stom-ach makes for a more comfortable night's sleep with a much lower risk of reflux. (Check out Chapter 6 for the complete scoop on diet and heartburn.)

Medicating nocturnal reflux

Chapter 10 has the lowdown on every conceivable prescription and over-the-counter (OTC) medicine for heartburn and reflux. Chapter 7 runs down the list of home remedies. For the purposes of this bedtime story, the important message is that any medicine or remedy that relieves heartburn during the day can also make you more comfortable at night.

Rolling the film on a good night's sleep

Oh, well, like Scarlett O'Hara in *Gone with the Wind,* you can think about that tomorrow. Tonight, when you finish this chapter, why not ease the way to dreamland with a good movie? Or with the quiz in the following table that asks you to match a Baker's Dozen — 13, count 'em, 13 — "sleep" movies to their movie stars. Psssst! Some of these films are a tad ancient.

Movie (Release Date)	Star(s)
1. The Big Sleep (1946)	a. Meg Ryan, Tom Hanks
2. The Big Sleep (1978)	b. Claudette Colbert, Robert Cummings
3. Sleeper (1973)	c. Eric Stolz, Meg Tilly
4. Sleepers (1996)	d. Julia Roberts
5. Sleeping Beauty (1959)	e. Simone Signoret, Yves Montand
6. The Sleeping Car Murder (1965)	f. Flora, Fauna, Merriweather, and Maleficent
7. Sleeping Dogs (1977)	g. Woody Allen, Diane Keaton
8. The Sleeping Tiger (1954)	h. Sam Neill
9. Sleep, My Love (1948)	i. Johnny Depp, Christina Ricci
10. Sleeping With the Enemy (1991)	j. Robert Mitchum, Sara Miles
11. Sleep With Me (1994)	k. Alexis Smith, Dirk Bogarde
12. Sleepless in Seattle (1993)	l. Kevin Bacon, Robert DeNiro, Dustin Hoffman
13. Sleepy Hollow (1999)	m. Lauren Bacall, Humphrey Bogart

Answers: *1. m; 2. j; 3. g; 4. l; 5. f; 6. e; 7. h; 8. k; 9. b; 10. d; 11. c; 12. a; 13. i*

Some medications are more potent than others. The most effective overall relief, including the most effective relief for nighttime heartburn, comes from *proton pump inhibitors* (PPI), the relatively new medicines that stop acid production at the source by quieting the glands in your stomach wall. This class of drugs includes esomeprazole (Nexium), lansoprazole (Prevacid), omeprazole (Prilosec, Prilosec OTC, Losec (Canada)), pantoprazole (Protonix), and rabeprazole (Aciphex).

Occasionally, people who don't get complete relief from a PPI may add another medication right before going to bed. If your heartburn is worse at night, you may feel better taking your PPI before your evening meal (dinner in the North, supper in the South), rather than before breakfast. But PPIs always work best when taken prior to a meal and work less well if you take them at bedtime.

Juggling drugs isn't a task for amateurs, so check with your doctor before playing doctor.

Chapter 15

Stressing Stress Relief

. . . .

In This Chapter

▶ Understanding how stress stresses

▶ Getting to know the adrenal glands

▶ Linking stress to heartburn

▶ Trying out some anti-stress techniques

. . . .

*L*ife is a roller coaster, up and down and up and down — and hopefully up again. You can't stop the bounce, but you can figure out ways to lessen its effects, especially the ones that hit on your gastrointestinal (GI) tract.

This chapter makes the connection between stress and heartburn/reflux, but I start out telling you how stress happens. I get to the good part — the link between stress and heartburn — after all that explanation. Got no patience? Skip ahead. But do yourself a favor and come back to read the other sections afterwards. The more you know, the less likely you are to hurt.

Stressing the Importance of Stress

Your boss, the mentor who hired and promoted you, has been fired. You go to pick up your new, incredibly expensive tweed jacket from the cleaner, and they can't find it. You walk into the coffee shop and see your significant other holding hands with someone else.

Your brain tells you to sit down, calm down, and relax. But, facing an imminent threat — you may be fired, too; an expensive garment's gone; your love's lost — your body goes into hyperdrive, pumping out hormones that pump you up, a physical reaction known as an *adrenal rush*. Your heart beats faster, you breathe deeper and quicker, and your muscles tense for "fight or flight," another name for that adrenal rush.

This, gentle reader, is stress with a capital *S,* and the National Heartburn Alliance (NHBA) says what most people with heartburn know: When stress strikes, reflux rises. To relieve your heartburn, you need to know how stress happens, how your body reacts, and how you can alleviate (if not totally control) the situation.

Activating Your Adrenals

Your adrenal glands are the humming hormone factories that power the stress reaction. Adrenals come as a couple, one atop each kidney (*ad* means *on* or *from; renal* means *kidney*). Each adrenal gland is a two-level structure with an outer covering, called the *adrenal cortex,* and an inner gland, called the *adrenal medulla.*

Both the adrenal cortex and the adrenal medulla respond to chemical signals from your *pituitary gland,* a small structure tucked into your brain pretty much in a straight line back from the bridge of your nose. When your body is stressed, the pituitary gland releases compounds that turn on your adrenal glands.

Considering the cortex

The adrenal cortex produces three kinds of hormones called *corticosteroids.* Under stress, your pituitary gland secretes higher amounts of corticotropin-releasing factor (CRF) to tell the adrenal cortex to increase its production of corticosteroids.

- ✔ **Androgens:** Male sex hormones, such as testosterone. You know what they do, right? If not, put this book down right now and go check out *Sex For Dummies* by Ruth K. Westheimer (Wiley).

- ✔ **Glucocorticoids:** Compounds that tell your liver to convert fat and protein to glucose and raise the level of sugar in your blood. The primary glucocorticoid is *cortisol,* a lead player in the stress reaction.

- ✔ **Mineralocorticoids:** Compounds that influence mineral metabolism. For example, the mineralocorticoid *aldosterone* regulates your body's sodium levels so that you can maintain normal blood pressure even when you're perspiring heavily or urinating frequently and losing a lot of salt.

Looking into the medulla

Pituitary hormones tell the adrenal medulla to release two important neurotransmitters:

- **Adrenaline:** Also called epinephrine
- **Noradrenaline:** Also known as norepinephrine

Neurotransmitters are chemicals that enable nerve cells to transmit messages back and forth. Ordinarily, neurotransmitters are released at a *synapse* — a place where two nerve cells talk to each other. But the adrenal neurotransmitters zip straight out into your bloodstream to circulate all around your body. And boy, the primary one, adrenaline, sure get things moving!

Getting ready for "fight or flight"

The release of cortisol and adrenaline into your body produces an effect similar to what happens when you toss an ice cube into a glass of carbonated soda: Things fizz up all over the place.

When good glands go bad

Every little organ has an illness all its own. The adrenal glands have two. The first is *Addison's disease,* in which the body doesn't produce enough corticosteroids, producing such symptoms as weakness, fatigue, low blood pressure, and intestinal upset. The second is *Cushing's syndrome,* in which the body churns out too much corticosteroids, leading to symptoms such as muscle weakness, thinning skin, easy bruising, and high blood pressure. Both illnesses are named for the men who discovered them — English physician Thomas Addison (1793–1860) and Boston neurosurgeon Harvey Cushing (1869–1939).

Addison's disease usually happens because of an attack by the body's immune system that destroys the adrenal gland, but it may also follow an adrenal infection. Either way, you can treat it with corticosteroid medicines. Cushing's syndrome may be due to a tumor of the adrenal gland or of the pituitary gland, or it may occur following the use of steroid drugs to treat arthritis or prevent rejection of a new organ after transplant. If the cause is a tumor, doctors can treat Cushing's syndrome surgically. If the cause is medication, you usually just need to have your doctor adjust your dosage.

Switches switch. Lights light. Connections connect. I'm speaking figuratively, of course, but under stress, your body really does seem to buzz with excitement, turning on defense systems and shutting down nonessential functions that may reduce your endurance or hinder your ability to fight — or run away and live to fight another day.

Does that sound dramatic? Absolutely. But even when you know that your crisis isn't life-threatening — you'll find another mentor; the cleaner will either find your jacket or pay for a substitute; and, although your heart may be broken, it keeps on beating — your body can't tell the difference. You have the same exact physical reaction, whether the crisis is dry-cleaning or a speeding bullet.

For a summary of your body's "fight or flight" responses, just run your finger down Table 15-1.

Table 15-1	Answering the Adrenals
Organ/System	*Effect of Adrenal Hormones*
Defense Systems (Increased Activity)	
Blood	Clots faster to reduce blood loss through injury.
Eyes	Pupils narrow to focus vision.
Heart	Beats faster; increases blood flow to skeletal muscles; sends more oxygen to every cell.
Lungs	Breathe faster and deeper to increase oxygen intake.
Muscles	Skeletal muscles tense in preparation for fight or flight.
Skin	Tenses to avoid injury.
Nonessential Systems	
Gastrointestinal tract	Contractions of stomach muscles slow as blood is diverted to skeletal muscles; digestion slows; food remains in stomach; contractions of colon increase to expel waste.
Immune system	Activity reduced to avoid reactions that may interfere with defense.
Reproductive system	Sexual responses diminish.
Urinary system	Urge to urinate suppressed.

Linking Stress to Heartburn

For most of us, the stress reaction ends when danger recedes. You get a new promotion, you get you jacket back, you find a new love, and your life returns more or less to normal.

But for some people, stress is a way of life. They may be dreadfully unlucky, with illness and crises piling up on top of each other. Or they may approach life at top speed, every day, all the time. Either way, their bodies are likely to respond uncomfortably to the constant bombardment of excess amounts of adrenal hormones. Table 15-2 lists some the problems that may arise in response to this continuous physical or emotional stress.

Table 15-2	Stress-Related Problems
Organ/System	*Possible Stress Reactions*
Heart/blood vessels	Angina, high blood pressure
Immune system	Allergies, asthma, respiratory illness
Intestinal tract	Spasm of intestinal muscles, leading to colitis or irritable bowel syndrome (IBS)
Skin	Acne, eczema, hives, pigment loss, psoriasis, rosacea
Muscles	Spasm leading to eyelid twitch, carpal tunnel syndrome, facial pain, headache, neck or back pain, TMJD (tempero-mandibular joint disorder)

When facing all the small stresses in life, different people approach the situation differently. For some people, the sound of chalk scratching across a blackboard is enough to trigger a migraine headache. For others, the chalk scratch is just another sound in the daily symphony. The Big Ones are different. Events such as the death of a spouse, the loss of a job, or being sentenced to prison are equally stressful to virtually everyone.

But the National Heartburn Alliance (NHBA) says that more than half of the people with heartburn feel worse when stressed. According to NHBA

✔ 52 percent of people with heartburn say the pain in their middle is related to stress at work.

✔ 58 percent of frequent heartburn sufferers identify "hectic lifestyle" — that lost jacket, that (sob!) faithless lover — as a heartburn trigger.

Given stress's effects on the gastrointestinal tract, who can blame them?

Hitting your GI tract with hormones

Your GI tract — described in detail in Chapter 2 — is essentially a long tube designed to move food efficiently through your body from one end (your mouth) to the other (your you-know-what).

The job is done via *peristalsis,* contractions of the muscular walls of each section of the tube: your esophagus, your stomach, your small intestine, and your large intestine. Anything that weakens these contractions slows the passage of food; anything that strengthens these contractions speeds up the process.

Would you believe that stress does both? Well, believe it! Under stress, hormones released by your pituitary gland and your adrenal glands

- ✔ Strengthen the contractions of your colon walls so that any waste present in your colon is expelled more quickly
- ✔ Weaken the contractions of your stomach walls so that any food present in your stomach stays there longer

The results are predictable. Under stress, people are more likely to develop diarrhea. And reflux.

The *lower esophageal sphincter* (LES) is a trapdoor between your esophagus and stomach that closes tight after you swallow to prevent acidic stomach contents from sliding backwards into the esophagus. But a full stomach presses up against the LES. The fuller the stomach and/or the longer the stomach stays full, the higher the pressure, and the greater the odds that the LES will pop open, allowing acidic stomach stuff to enter the esophagus and cause heartburn. Ouch.

Bodies behaving badly

Hormones aren't the only reason stress increases the risk of reflux. Your behavior also counts. Under stress, you find it easy to say, or think, something like, "Things are so bad, how much worse can it be if I say to heck with the rules and do things I never do like smoking and drinking a lot and eating foods I know upset my stomach?"

But when stress strikes, your body deserves tender loving care, not a leap off the Heartburn Cliffs. The fact is that anything that lit your heartburn in ordinary times is *much* more likely to do so now.

So give your esophagus a break. Eventually, the current stress will end. Until it does, find a constructive way to reduce — or at least cope with — your stress. Check out the mind-body therapy methods listed in the very next section. It may just work for you. Or maybe not. To put it mildly, the research is iffy.

Unlocking Your Stomach from Your Stress

Any technique that uses the power of your mind to produce changes in your body can be defined as *mind-body therapy*. The mother of all mind-body therapies is *meditation*, the ancient process that advocates concentration as a path to relaxation. The major modern mind-body therapy is psychoanalysis, created by Sigmund Freud and modified by dozens of disciples ever since. The newest entries are technologically oriented regimens such as biofeedback and imagery.

Mind-body therapies certainly have their differences. Meditation says, "Go into yourself for contentment." Psychoanalysis says, "Look inside — but analyze for change." Biofeedback says, "Use the physical energy of your brain to alter body processes." But all share the conviction that how and what you think can be a force for change — like removing the triggers that lead to reflux.

Examining antireflux anti-stress therapy

After you know stress makes heartburn burn more fiercely, the natural question is "What anti-stress therapy will work for me?"

Every mother knows the simple answer: Clean your closets. Paint your house. Walk the dog. But Dr. Mom probably has no scientific studies to prove her case. So when the U.S. Department of Health and Human Services' Agency for Healthcare Research and Quality (AHRQ) released its *Evidence Report/Technology Assessment No. 40, Mind-Body Interventions for Gastrointestinal Conditions* in March 2001, closet cleaning and house painting weren't on the list. Table 15-3 shows some of the therapies AHRQ included.

Table 15-3	AHRQ's List of Mind-Body Therapies
Therapy	*What It Is*
Behavioral therapy	A form of conditioning used to alter behavior. For example, if you're afraid of snakes, the behavioral therapist, usually a psychologist, may ask you to visit the reptile house at the local zoo every day for a week to condition you to snakes and thus reduce your fear.
Biofeedback	A technique that seeks to teach you how to control the functions of the autonomic nervous system, such as heartbeat, respiration, and body temperature.

(continued)

Table 15-3 *(continued)*

Therapy	What It Is
Cognitive therapy	The collective name for processes that use imaging and self-discovery to change the body.
Imagery (guided)	A therapy which suggests that you can relieve anxiety or pain by teaching yourself to visualize calming alternatives during a painful or stressful situation, such as childbirth.
Hypnosis	An artificially induced trancelike state during which the hypnotist offers suggestions (like cigarettes taste awful) that remain in the mind after the patient has returned to a conscious state. A medical hypnotist is a doctor with training in hypnosis.
Meditation	A form of mild self-hypnosis intended to provide relaxation from anxiety or pain. The best-known form is Transcendental Meditation.
Placebo therapy	A therapy based on the power of suggestion in which a nonmedical product or treatment (such as a look-alike "sugar" pill or a dummy incision) is used rather than actual medicine or surgery to provide relief.
Multi-modal therapy	A little of this therapy, a little of that — the scientific equivalent of, "Hey, whatever works."

Reading the AHRQ report

Digging its way through a list of online medical research databases, such as MEDLine, AHRQ came up with a total of 53 studies of the therapies listed in Table 15-3. Carefully reviewing the studies, the agency concluded that

✔ Studies on the effects of mind/body techniques for GI problems aren't yet totally reliable because of structural problems, such as a number of volunteers too small to provide hard data.

✔ Biofeedback has been the subject of the greatest number of mind/body therapy studies for GI conditions with 17. The results are mixed, meaning sometimes it works and sometimes it doesn't.

✔ The runners-up include hypnosis (8 studies), relaxation therapy (8), behavioral therapy (8), multimodal therapy (4), cognitive therapy (4), imagery (2), and placebo (1). The results in these studies are also mixed.

Considering these conclusions, AHRQ then did what any self-respecting research group would do with such inconclusive results. It recommended trying again in the future when it may have access to more and better studies — and maybe more data on the value of closet cleaning and house painting.

While you're waiting, you can read the report — AHRQ Publication No. 01-E027 — for yourself:

- ✔ **Online:** hstat.nlm.nih.gov/hq/Hquest/screen/DirectAccess/db/3703
- ✔ **Download:** www.ahrq.gov/clinic/evrptfiles.htm#mindbod
- ✔ **Print copy (free):** 800-358-9295

Finding a solution

The bad news from the AHRQ report is that that mind/body techniques have no proven scientific record of success in relieving reflux-related heartburn. The good news is that the studies probably didn't include you, an individual with your particular body and your particular stress reactions.

Remember the stress list that started this chapter? You know — losing your mentor, losing your jacket, and losing your love. For some people, these situations are Atomic Level Crises; for others, simply a sign that the body really needs chocolate. As a result, no study (not even an Official Government Report) can tell you for sure whether an anti-stress technique can help relieve your stress. How well you do on any therapy may also be a function of your general health, your general attitude, and maybe plain, old-fashioned determination.

Dr. Schuster's biofeedback story

Dr. Marvin Schuster, a psychiatrist and gastroenterologist at Johns Hopkins, must be one heck of a determined guy. In 1974, when he decided to test biofeedback as a method for controlling reflux, Schuster picked a volunteer he knew very well: Himself.

To do his study on himself, he slid a narrow tube through his nose and down his throat all the way to his LES, the trapdoor between esophagus and stomach which prevents stomach contents from flowing back (refluxing) into the throat.

Schuster's catheter had a gauge on the end to measure pressure at the LES and display it on a meter, so that Schuster could see what happened when he attempted to contract and relax the LES. Eventually, Schuster succeeded, learning to keep his LES closed after swallowing and thus reduce his risk of reflux. Wow.

Choosing an anti-stress technique

The only way to know whether an anti-stress technique will work for you is to try it. Just pick a therapy that sounds friendly, find a book, class, or practitioner, and give it a whirl. If it works, good. If it doesn't, try something else. Table 15-4 gives you a list of sources for details on mind/body anti-stress techniques.

These sources not only provide an overview of the relevant discipline, they also give you access to a list of professionals. However, never hand your body (or your mind) to any practitioner without first checking with your own doctor. And always check every professional's credentials; state medical societies, listed in Chapter 8, are a good place to start.

Table 15-4	Web Sites on Anti-Stress Techniques
Technique	**Organization Web Site**
Behavioral therapy	Association for the Advancement of Behavior Therapy; Web site `www.aabt.org`
Biofeedback	The Association for Applied Psychophysiology and Biofeedback (AAPB); Web site `www.aapb.org`
Hypnosis	American Society for Clinical Hypnosis; Web site `www.asch.net`
Meditation	The Transcendental Meditation Program; Web site `www.tm.org`
Psychoanalysis	American Psychiatric Association; Web site `www.psych.org`

Remembering the tried and true

In Chapter 13, you can read about using exercise to build a better, stronger body. You can also use exercise as a relaxation technique that slows your heartbeat, increases your respiration, and just plain takes your mind off what ails you (always a good strategy when stress strikes). You know, like cleaning closets and painting houses — both can count as exercise, and they offer extra benefits (you can find your clothes, the house looks better).

As Chapter 13 says, avoid exercises that turn you upside down or twist you into a pretzel. Both positions may put pressure on your LES, thus increasing rather than lowering your risk of reflux. No standing on your head. No wrapping your ankles around your ears. As little bending from the waist as possible. No running: A weak LES may pop open when you bounce up and down.

If all else fails, move!

Urban Centers of Heartburn Heck are cities, towns, and villages named in a 2003 National Heartburn Alliance (NHBA) survey as the places with a much higher-than-normal number of people suffering from reflux-related heartburn. Strangely enough, even though NHBA reports that stress can cause heartburn, that list of high-heartburn cities in Chapter 4 doesn't correlate with the list of the Ten Most Stressful Cities published by *Money* magazine in January 2004. Go figure.

In any event, to make the *Money* magazine stressful list, a city must rack up high numbers in such miserable categories as divorce, suicide, and unemployment, stress enough for anybody. How high is "high"? This high. These statistics from Tacoma, Washington, America's Number One Stress City in 2004, say it all:

- The divorce rate is sky-high, up in the 95th percentile among American cities.

- The suicide rate is equally astronomical, in the 92nd percentile.

- The unemployment rate hit 7.7 percent, nearly two points higher than the national average.

Is it any wonder people living in the following cities spend a lot of time shopping for antacids?

- Tacoma, Washington

- Miami, Florida

- New Orleans, Louisiana

- Las Vegas, Nevada

- New York, New York

- Portland, Oregon

- Mobile, Alabama

- Stockton-Lodi, California

- Detroit, Michigan

- Dallas, Texas

How do you spell geographical relief? According to *Money* magazine, the state-capital zones of Albany-Schenectady-Troy in New York State and Harrisburg-Lebanon-Carlisle in Pennsylvania are tied for the Least Stressful title. Other low-stress sites include laid-back Orange County, California; suburban Nassau-Suffolk counties, New York; and Minneapolis-St. Paul, Minnesota.

Chapter 16

Fashioning (and Furnishing) a Comfortable Life

This short but useful chapter covers two topics that may seem to be an odd couple. Just call them the Two F's — fashion and furniture — and see how handling them well can help keep your reflux at bay.

Your foray into fashion begins with an explanation of how some superstylish clothes may unstylishly increase your risk of heartburn. Next, I zero in on cosmetics and makeup. Sad to say, sometimes just a sniff of an irritating ingredient or product may be enough to trigger heartburn — even if you're not the one wearing the pretty stuff. This chapter provides pointers on how to cope.

After you look good, you want to be comfortable, right? So I also focus on home furnishings, explaining why where you sit and sleep can play an important but often-overlooked role in helping to reduce your risk of heartburn. Which chair? What bed? Read on to find out.

Burning Your Bra and Loosening Your Belt

Take a deep breath. No, a *really* deep breath. Feel what happens? Your chest juts out and you feel a slight lift as all the organs in the middle of your body move up. What you're experiencing is an event known scientifically as *an increase in intra-abdominal pressure.* Now imagine holding that position for several hours at a time.

Everyone wants to look slim and trim — especially when special occasions call for slipping into that special dress, stylish skirt, trendy suit, or hip black tux. But for people with heartburn, the price of reining in your body with tight clothes is higher than you might expect. When you put on tight clothes and cinch in your middle, you increase the pressure on your middle, which increases the pressure on your lower esophageal sphincter (LES), which increases the possibility that the LES (that trapdoor between stomach and esophagus) may accidentally open, allowing acid stomach contents to flow back into the esophagus.

Result? Heartburn. To avoid the pain, you want to relax tight

- ✔ Belts
- ✔ Bras
- ✔ Bustiers
- ✔ Corsets
- ✔ Garter belts
- ✔ Girdles
- ✔ Jeans so snug you have to lie down on the bed to zip them — Oooof
- ✔ Pantyhose
- ✔ Waist-cinchers

Chapter 17 explains how being pregnant also pushes the stomach up against the LES, especially if a woman avoids maternity clothes with a stretchy waist. Chapter 13 explains why having fat around the middle (beer belly) may also trigger heartburn. Furthermore, if you have a backache, wearing an elastic brace too tight for your body may lead to the same result.

A word about Thomas King Chambers (1818–1889)

More than a century ago, a British doctor, Thomas King Chambers, made a name for himself by pinning some female digestive problems squarely on corsets, known familiarly as *bodies,* presumably shorthand for *bodices.* Putting on a corset, said Chambers, "dragged and pushed" the female stomach heaven-knows-where. Unfortunately, Chambers' discovery that a girl's desire to turn herself into an hourglass can be unpleasantly uncomfortable didn't secure him a place in the major histories of medicine. But his *magnum opus* (Latin for *Big Work*), titled *The Indigestions; Or Diseases of the Digestive Organs Functionally Treated,* lives on. You can find it on www.google.com — and that's probably as close to immortality as anyone might wish!

If you suffer from heartburn, the time has come to make a healthier and happier fashion statement. Toss out *Vogue.* Cancel your subscriptions to *Harper's Bazaar, Details, GQ,* and all the other fashionista rags. If you have heartburn, take your second deep breath of this chapter and admit that a snappy outfit may be a boon to the spirit, but not at the price of a pain in the middle.

Does that mean you have to forget fashion to appease your digestive tract? Good heavens, no. Just remember the Golden Rule and do unto your digestive tract what you would have it do unto you: Give it some space and take some of the following precautions:

✔ **Buy the right size:** Grit your teeth, square your shoulders, march into your favorite store, and pick a waist size that fits. If it absolutely, totally drives you nuts to wear a size larger than you're used to, cut the tag out of your old clothes and sew it into the new stuff. Every time you look, you'll see the size that makes you happy.

This advice also applies to garments, such as girdles and garter belts, that are supposed to be tight. If you buy a slightly larger size, you can achieve a smooth line under your clothes without squeezing your body so tight that you're uncomfortable. When in doubt, aim for a more comfortable situation. Your reward? Less risk of reflux-related heartburn.

✔ **Dress for dinner:** Don't wear tight stuff when you sit down to dinner. Or — don't tell anyone — just quietly open the top button. No one will ever notice.

✔ **Give up belts:** Try suspenders instead. Red ones — or not.

✔ **Pass up elastic waistbands:** Yes, elastic is, well, elastic which means it stretches. But the stretched waistband is still tight — and the elastic keeps exerting pressure to revert to its original size. In other words, a stretched elastic waistband is still too tight for comfort.

Looking Good, Feeling Fine

Cosmetics and heartburn? Yes, the link's a stretch, but it does connect through allergic reactions. Lots of ingredients may trigger your allergies, but according to the North American Contact Dermatitis Group, perfumes — sometimes listed as *fragrance* — are the prime offenders.

You can read about the study, considered a classic, in the November 1986 issue of *FDA Consumer,* the person-friendly periodical available free from the Food and Drug Administration. To find it online, log on `www.fda.gov`. When the home page appears, type "Cosmetic Allergies 1986" into the search bar. Bingo! Ain't technology grand?

Running down perfume's effects

If you're sensitive to perfume, you know what it does to your body. When you put some on or when you're within sniffing distance of someone using the smelly stuff

- ✔ Your eyes may itch.
- ✔ Your nose may run.
- ✔ You may sneeze.
- ✔ You may develop a postnasal drip as liquid leaking from your irritated tissues trickles down your throat.

And therein lies the link to heartburn. As Chapter 4 explains, respiratory problems leading to coughing and clearing your throat are common reflux triggers. To avoid the perfume and the trigger, you may spend a lot of time checking cosmetic labels for some indication that the product is made without perfume. But can you trust the labels? Probably not.

Questioning the accuracy of cosmetic label terms

People with allergies often look for the word _hypoallergenic_ on the label before they plunk down their hard-earned cash for a beautifying product. That logic certainly sounds smart. After all, when the dictionary says that _hypo-_ means _less_, you're entitled to assume that _hypoallergenic_ means _less likely to cause allergies_. Unfortunately, it isn't necessarily so.

Protecting animals

Add the terms _cruelty-free_ and _not tested on animals_ to your list of suspect label claims. As the FDA explains, many raw materials used in cosmetics were tested on animals years ago when they were first introduced.

Although some cosmetic companies may now use scientific literature, nonanimal testing, or controlled human-use testing to make sure their products are safe, others may be applying feel-good, anticruelty phrases to finished products, such as shampoo, lipstick, mascara, or whatever, and not to the specific ingredients.

If using cosmetics made without animal testing is your personal line in the sand, don't take the label on faith. Get the facts, in writing, from the manufacturer. And if the company waffles, tell 'em they're toast.

Despite decades of trying, the FDA has never been able to establish standards for what constitutes a hypoallergenic cosmetic product. Every time the agency proposes something, the various cosmetic companies sprint into one court or another, and darned if they don't get the proposal tossed out.

So right now the word *hypoallergenic* means whatever the manufacturer wants. For one company that may translate as avoiding perfume; for another, it may mean skipping some irritating coloring agents. As a result, the only way to be certain that a product doesn't trigger your allergies (and perhaps your reflux) is to try it. Bummer.

By the way, *hypoallergenic* isn't the only undefined cosmetic label term. Some others include

- *Allergy-tested* (What allergy? Which test?)
- *Dermatologist-tested* (What dermatologist? Which test?)
- *Fragrance-free* (Even with this on the package, a cosmetic may contain small amounts of perfume to mask other odors.)
- *Nonirritating* (To what? Or to whom?)
- *Sensitivity-tested* (Whose sensitivity? Which test?)

Two cosmetic label terms with real meaning are *natural* and *non-comedogenic*.

- The word *natural* on a cosmetic label tells you the product is made with ingredients that come from plants or animal products rather than from an ingredient made in a laboratory. Does that guarantee safety or rule out an allergic reaction? No, because *natural* doesn't always mean *okey-dokey*. Arsenic, after all, is both a natural substance and darned deadly poison, while lanolin, a natural moisturizer from the wool of sheep, is a proven allergen.
- *Non-comedogenic* is more reliable. True, no federal standard exists for the term, but non-comedogenic products generally don't contain ingredients that can clog your pores (boooo!) and lead to acne (ugh!).

Finding the facts on ingredients and label terms

Want to know more about a specific cosmetic ingredient or label term? Well, you can search the Internet for every ingredient on every label in your cosmetics cabinet. Or you can log on the FDA Center for Food Safety and Applied Nutrition's cosmetics page (no, I have no idea why FDA lists cosmetics under a food and nutrition heading), www.cfsan.fda.gov/~dms/cos-prd.html.

Another good source is science writer Ruth Winter's *A Consumer's Dictionary of Cosmetic Ingredients* (Crown), an authoritative guide to more than 5,000 ingredients.

Reducing reactions to cosmetics

All cosmetics contain either natural or synthetic preservatives to protect them from the inevitable contamination that occurs when you open a bottle or touch something like lipstick to your skin.

Time out. *Preservative* isn't a dirty word. In fact, just the opposite. Preservatives prevent the growth of harmful microorganisms, such as molds and bacteria, thus keeping your cosmetics safe. Before they're sold to cosmetics makers for use in cosmetics, preservatives and other cosmetic ingredients have been tested for safety. And guess what? Some preservatives, such as citric acid (the compound that makes citrus fruits tart), are natural.

After you get your makeup home, your task is to treat your cosmetics with tender, loving care so as to minimize the growth of molds that can make you sneeze and drip (increasing your risk of heartburn), or bugs that can cause infections (increasing your risk of, well, infections). The following are a few simple do's and don'ts:

- Do keep makeup in a cool dark place, protected from heat and sunlight that can break down protective preservatives.

- Do rotate your cosmetics every six months. Old cosmetics — especially liquids — are potential bug factories.

  Bacteria and mold need water to survive, so dry products such as cosmetic powders are likely to stay safer longer than liquid-based lotions and creams.

- Don't use eye makeup when you have an eye infection. (Throw out any product you used before you knew you had the infection.)

- Don't add water to a product to "stretch" the product. Water dilutes the preservatives.

- Don't moisten cosmetics with saliva. Yes, Chapter 3 says that saliva is a natural antacid that neutralizes stomach acid, but that saliva is flowing naturally down your esophagus, and the fact that it carries multitudes of germs that live — naturally — in your mouth doesn't matter. Adding saliva to cosmetics may turn them into germ soup.

- Don't share cosmetics. Not even with your best friend or your daughter. Who knows what she has that you don't?

What's a cosmetic, anyway?

The Federal Food, Drug, and Cosmetic Act defines *cosmetics* as "articles other than soap, which are applied to the human body for cleansing, beautifying, promoting attractiveness, or altering the appearance." The FDA list includes (in the appropriate alphabetical order): Baby products, bath oils and bubble baths, deodorants, eye makeup, fragrances, hair coloring, hair cleansers and conditioners (shampoo, conditioners, curling and straightening products, shiners, volumizers, and so one), manicure products, makeup other than eye makeup (lipstick, foundation, blush, and so on), skin-care products (creams, lotions, powders, sprays), and tanning products.

Finding Furniture That Fights Heartburn

Standing is easy on the digestive tract. When you're upright, everything goes right where it's supposed to be, lessening your risk of heartburn. But when you sit or lie down, all heck can break loose.

Picking a proper chair

Sitting seems like such a simple task, doesn't it? But if you're forced to bend your body to conform to the chair, couch, or recliner in question, you may end up with a reflux reaction.

To visualize the perfect chair for people with heartburn, close your eyes and think "Shaker." Straight back. Square seat. Just the right height so that your feet meet the floor square on. The Shaker chair, like other Shaker products, was created to show the beauty of simplicity. The bonus is its ability to let your digestive organs sit right where they're supposed to be (as you can see in Figure 16-1). Now imagine yourself curling into a recliner or an oversize plush armchair at the end of a long, hard day. Feel your backbone curving as you slide down into the pillows? Feel yourself turning into one great big ol' letter *C*?

When you don't sit up straight, your stomach can push up against your esophagus (see the second illustration in Figure 16-1), increasing the likelihood that your LES will open, letting those acidic stomach contents flow back and produce heartburn. You may adore plushy stuff, or slouching in your seat, but just think back to how happy your digestive tract looks in the first illustration in Figure 16-1.

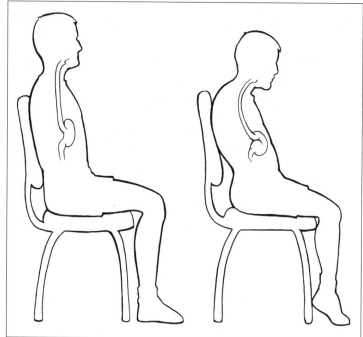

Figure 16-1:
Keeping
things
straight.

And don't you think that sitting up straight while eating to keep your digestive tract in a straight line down from your mouth to your tummy is a really good idea? You bet it is.

Making your bed for a good night's sleep

Nighttime heartburn is fairly common (as I discuss in Chapters 3). Why is night so conducive to heartburn? To find the answer, bookmark this page and turn back to Chapter 2 to peruse the diagram of your digestive tract.

As you plainly can see, your eating-and-excreting system is a long tube that runs from mouth to, well, the other end of your body. After you look at the picture, think about what happens when you lie down to sleep. (Or sneak a peak at the figures in Chapter 14 that detail the layout of your digestive tract when you sleep in various positions.)

- ✔ If you lie flat, your digestive tube also is flat, and whatever is in your stomach can just slide back through the LES to irritate your esophagus.

- ✔ But if you elevate your head, the acid stuff in your stomach is more likely to stay where it belongs.

See the difference? But, how to achieve a comfortable version of position number two? No problem; it's a furniture thing.

Meeting a mattress

Your mattress is the platform on which you build a good night's sleep. The basic choice when comparing mattresses is hard or soft. If your mattress if too soft, your body will bend in the middle like a big U.

Yes, your head is higher than your middle, but so are your legs. Spend a night in this contorted position, and the next morning you'll have so many aches and pains in so many new and unexpected places that you won't have time to worry about heartburn.

The better choice is almost certainly a medium-firm or firm mattress that gives you enough support to lie flat. After you have that straight, you can concentrate on positioning your upper body to keep your esophagus comfortably above your tummy.

Creating an incline

You have a number of options to elevate your head above your esophagus, and thus let gravity help you keep the acidic stomach contents in your stomach and out of your esophagus. Some are better than others. You can pile up pillows behind your head, but doing that produces a steep angle that can give you a crick in the neck.

I suggest taking one of these approaches (which you check out in Figure 16-2):

- ✔ Insert a riser under the back legs of your bed to lift the head of your bed about six inches higher than the foot. If you take this route, be sure to secure the riser to the bed frame. I don't know about you, but I can see myself leaping into bed and bringing the whole thing crashing down on the floor.

- ✔ If you're the only one in your bed, you can try sticking one regular pillow or a wedge-shape pillow under the mattress to build a sloping incline. Of course, if you have a partner, his or her side of the bed will be a tad uneven, but love involves sacrifice, right? In any event, whether you choose firm feathers or firm synthetic foam, the rise will be smooth and gradual, starting at just below your shoulders. Put a pleasantly soft regular pillow on top of the mattress, and you may find yourself dreaming your way through the night without a heartburn twinge.

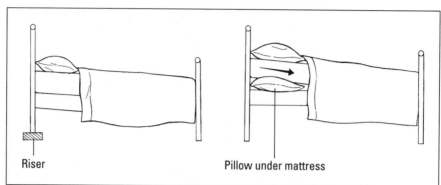

Figure 16-2:
Rising to the
occasion.   Riser   Pillow under mattress

Bed and back

For years, orthopedists have told people with lower back pain to sleep on firm mattresses, but a recent 313-person study published in *Lancet,* the British medical journal, says, "Phooey to that!"

In the study led by Dr. Francisco Kovacs of the Kovacs Foundation, Paseo Mallorca, Palma de Mallorca, Spain, volunteers with lower-back pain were randomly assigned to sleep on a firm mattress or a medium-firm one for 90 nights.

In the end (as well as in the lower back), the medium-firm beds were the clear winners. People sleeping in them were two times more likely than people sleeping on firm mattresses to say, "I feel better when I get up in the morning, I feel better all day, and I feel better when I lie down at night." The only glitch in the survey was that nobody asked the patients whether just being in gorgeous Mallorca made them feel better.

Part V
Meeting the Special Cases

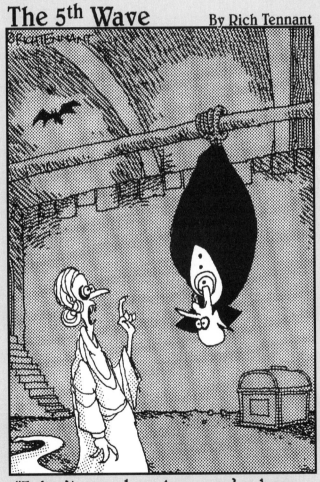

The 5th Wave   By Rich Tennant

"I don't care how long you've been sleeping like that, I still think it's contributing to your reflux problem."

In this part . . .

Pregnant women, infants and children, and older people are folks who may need specific help to identify their heartburn symptoms and prevent their reflux. This part tells you in exact detail which symptoms affect what group and which remedies work for whom.

Chapter 17

Handling the Heartburn of Pregnancy

. . . .

In This Chapter

▶ Deciding who's at risk

▶ Staying away from unneeded tests

▶ Evaluating drugs for pregnant women

▶ Changing your lifestyle to match your changing body

. . . .

First off, let me say, "Congratulations!" If you're perusing this chapter, I'm guessing that you or someone close to you is expecting — a baby that is. But you may or may not be aware that many expectant mothers can also expect to experience heartburn in the months leading up to the big day.

The discomfort from reflux may be the same in both pregnant women and non-pregnant women, but when a doctor treats a pregnant woman, he also treats her fetus, a situation that may affect decisions about diagnostic tests and anti-heartburn meds.

This chapter tells you why reflux is so common during pregnancy, explains how to recognize the symptoms, and lists ways to soothe the heartburn that so often seems an integral part of being pregnant. By the way, I make a larger-than-usual number of references to other chapters because some of the subjects in this chapter, such as what to avoid eating while pregnant, are covered in greater detail elsewhere for the general reader.

Are All Pregnant Women at Risk for Reflux?

I start with the good news. Having heartburn while you're pregnant is very uncomfortable, but it's rarely serious. On the other hand, being pregnant can raise absolute heck with the ol' gastrointestinal tract. Not only do many women experience the frequent nausea and vomiting called "morning sickness," but a majority also suffer from reflux and heartburn.

About 10 percent of women who aren't pregnant say they have heartburn at least once a day. But that number of daily sufferers bounces all the way up to 25 percent among pregnant women. And another 50 percent of expectant mothers experience at least an occasional twinge. Add it up, and you see that about 75 percent of pregnant women suffer from heartburn at one time or another through the course of their pregnancy

But life isn't exactly fair, and some pregnant women are more likely than others to experience heartburn. Who's most likely to develop reflux while pregnant?

- ✔ Women who have reflux before they get pregnant
- ✔ Women who have heartburn the first time they get pregnant (sorry, the experts say it only gets worse with subsequent pregnancies)
- ✔ Women who are carrying more than one baby — twins, triplets, and counting

Pregnancy increases your risk of reflux for two reasons. Being pregnant

- ✔ Changes the size and alters the position of your internal organs
- ✔ Changes your hormone production

Altering your insides

Ordinarily, the uterus (womb) is a small organ about the size of a pear, which as you can see in Illustration A in Figure 17-1, sits a bit below the belly button, well below the stomach, which normally rests in the upper part of the torso, nestled right behind the left ribs. ("Right" behind your "left" ribs? Oh, well . . .) But as Illustrations B and C in Figure 17-1 demonstrate, the pregnant uterus pushes up against the stomach.

When the uterus pushes against the stomach, the stomach, in turn, pushes up against the *diaphragm*. As a result, muscles in this area may weaken, creating a gap called a *hiatus* (more about that in Chapter 4), a small opening through which a bit of the stomach may squeeze up into the chest cavity, creating a *hiatal hernia*. The hiatal hernia pushes against the lower esophageal sphincter (LES) and, as Chapter 2 explains, the LES may open a bit, allowing acidic stomach contents to slip back into the esophagus. Result? Heartburn.

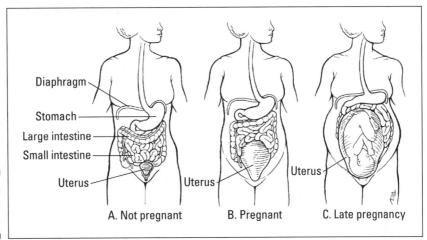

Figure 17-1:
A changing
female body.

Diaphragm
Stomach
Large intestine
Small intestine
Uterus

A. Not pregnant

Uterus
B. Pregnant

Uterus
C. Late pregnancy

In Chapter 2, you can find a detailed description of how reflux happens when your LES, the "trapdoor" from your stomach to your esophagus, opens at the wrong time, letting acidic stomach contents flow back into the more delicate esophagus.

Redecorating the baby's room

A healthy female body happily houses the woman who owns it. But when she becomes pregnant, a woman's body goes through a series of alterations designed to accommodate a tenant — the developing fetus. In addition to the gastrointestinal changes I detail in the "Altering your insides" section in this chapter, a whole host of other home repair and improvements take place:

✔ A pregnant woman produces extra blood.

✔ Her blood vessels relax, expanding to carry the blood to the fetus.

✔ Her heart beats faster, pumping out more blood each time her heart contracts in a beat.

✔ Late in pregnancy, as her uterus presses against her *vena cava* — the primary artery leading from the heart — she pumps out less blood per beat.

✔ She breathes faster, and her body stores more oxygen.

✔ Her skin and the *areola* (puckered skin around the nipple) may darken, and she may develop the "mask of pregnancy," a blotchy pigmented area across her cheeks and nose.

And then, when the baby is born, virtually all these changes disappear — until it's time for another tenant.

For more about healthcare and body changes during pregnancy, check out *Pregnancy For Dummies,* 2nd Edition, by Drs. Joanne Stone and Keith Eddelman (Wiley).

Raging hormones

The female sex hormones estrogen and progesterone are vital to a woman's reproductive health.

At puberty, estrogen

- Stimulates the maturation of the female reproductive organs
- Triggers the development of secondary sexual characteristics (breasts, body hair)
- Regulates menstruation and triggers the release of an egg each month from the ovaries

Anticipating the egg's fertilization by a passing sperm, progesterone, the second female hormone

- Prevents the release of a second egg
- Thickens and firms the walls of the uterus
- Nourishes blood vessels that will support the fetus (if the egg isn't fertilized, progesterone stimulates the shedding of the uterine walls that produce menstrual bleeding)

During pregnancy, estrogen and progesterone act as natural muscle relaxants, enabling the muscular walls of the uterus to expand to make room for the fetus. That's the good news. The bad news is that these hormones may trigger reflux and heartburn by relaxing muscle tissue in other parts of the body, leading to reflux and heartburn. What muscles? These muscles:

- **The LES:** The opening from the esophagus to the stomach, which usually shuts tight after swallowing to prevent acidic stomach contents from flowing back into the esophagus, may not close as tightly as it should or may open inadvertently from time to time. (See Chapter 2 for more about how the LES functions.)
- **The esophagus:** The muscular walls of the esophagus may not contract forcefully enough to push reflux material back into the stomach.
- **The stomach:** The muscular walls of the stomach may not contract strongly enough to move food efficiently into the small intestine. A full stomach pushes up against the hiatus.
- **The small and large intestines:** The muscular walls of the small and large intestines may not contract strongly enough to move food as quickly as usual through the digestive tract. Result? No, not reflux. This time the result is constipation, another digestion-related side effect of pregnancy.

What's in a name?

Possibly more than you want to know, but take a look anyway.

The female body makes three principal forms of estrogen: *Estradiol, estriol,* and *estrone.* Estradiol is the most potent member of the trio, and for scientists, the word *estrogen* actually means a form of estradiol called 17-b estrodiol.

Progesterone is the female hormone produced naturally in the body. Natural and synthetic chemicals that act like progesterone are called *progestogens.* The family name for progesterone and progestogens is *progestins,* the term sometimes used for the progestogens in birth control pills.

All clear?

Avoiding Unnecessary Tests

When you're pregnant, simply listing your symptoms may be enough to convince your doctor that you have reflux. Being able to effectively communicate your reflux-like symptoms to your doctor is important. Make a detailed list of your symptoms before your appointment so that you can paint a clear picture.

Read the following nutshell explanation of two common tests doctors generally avoid when a woman is pregnant.

- ✔ **Endoscopy:** As you can see in Chapter 9, endoscopy is a procedure that requires a specially trained doctor called an endoscopist to insert a slim tubelike instrument called an endoscope into your throat so she can examine the tissue. To do this, the doctor must give you a sedative — safe for you, but not necessarily for your baby.

  Doctors don't routinely recommend an endoscopy for pregnant women because it has the potential to harm the fetus. But, a doctor may occasionally believe that the benefit of knowing what's going on in a patient's digestive tract outweighs that risk. Clearly, the decision whether to use endoscopy is made one patient at a time.

- ✔ **X-rays:** A second common diagnostic test, the "barium swallow," requires you to drink a solution that a doctor can then visualize on X-rays of your torso. The barium solution, opaque on X-ray, shows up any defects in the upper digestive tract. Doctors rarely use this test because it exposes the fetus to radiation.

Given the fact that pregnancy-related reflux is a temporary discomfort that disappears after the baby makes his or her grand debut, you won't be surprised to discover that most doctors try to avoid unnecessary testing for reflux. Chapter 9 lists a bunch of other tests. Very few pregnant women undergo any of these tests or even the two previously listed. Most of the tests are probably safe, but why take a chance?

Determining Safe Remedies

All drugs have risks as well as benefits. Ordinarily the adverse effects affect only the person who takes the medicine. But when a woman is pregnant, a doctor must balance the benefits to the patient in front of him with the risks to the patient she's carrying.

To do that, doctors and patients must know

- ✓ Whether the drug crosses the placenta and reaches the fetus.

- ✓ Whether the drug can cause physical malformations in the developing fetus. In science-speak, chemicals and drugs that cause physical damage are called *teratogens* (from the Greek word roots *teras* meaning *monster* and *gen* meaning *make*).

- ✓ Whether the drug damages genes and chromosomes. Science-speak for this sort of substance is *mutagen*.

How's a person supposed to navigate such a seemingly complex path? Not to worry. The hoofbeats you hear in the distance are the sound of the Food and Drug Administration (FDA) good guys riding to the rescue.

Reviewing the ABCs of drugs for pregnant women

In 1979, the FDA came up with the first system used to quantify a drug's potential to injure a fetus physically or damage its genes and chromosomes.

The system — still in use — places every drug sold in the United States into one of five risk categories: A, B, C, D, or X.

Category A

These drugs have gone through well-controlled scientific studies with pregnant women and show no risk to the fetus. The FDA believes there is only a remote possibility that Category A drugs will injure a developing fetus. Liothyuronine, a thyroid hormone product, is an example of a Category A drug.

Category B

These drugs have tested safe for animal fetuses, but no well-controlled studies with pregnant women have been conducted.

> *Or*

Category B drugs may have injured animal fetuses, but studies with pregnant women don't show any problems with human fetuses.

Metronidazole (Flagyl), an anti-infective used to treat yeast infections, is an example of a Category B drug.

Category C

These drugs have damaged fetuses in tests with pregnant animals, but no studies with pregnant women have been conducted.

> *Or*

No adequate data from either animal or human studies exists, **and** in some cases, the benefits of the drug may be more important than its potential risks.

The minimally sedating antihistamines astemizole (Hismanal), desloratadine (Clarinex), fexofenadine (Allegra), and loratadine (Claritin) are examples of Category C drugs.

Category D

These drugs are considered hazardous to human fetuses based on human studies or on incidents reported before or after the drug went on sale. Pregnant women should only use these drugs in life-threatening situations for which no other remedy exists. The tranquilizer lorazepam (Ativan) is an example of a Category D drug.

Category X

These drugs have damaged fetuses in both animal and human studies.

> *Or*

There have been reports of damage before or after the drug went on sale indicating serious human fetal injury or death.

Down Under with Australian alternatives

The FDA's ABCs are useful enough to have been adopted in other countries, sometimes with minor changes to make them more precise predictors of drug safety. For example, in Australia and New Zealand, Category B — drugs that may have harmed some animal fetuses but have been tested and proved safe in human beings — mutates into three categories:

✔ **Category B1:** Drugs have been taken by only a limited number of pregnant women and women of childbearing age with no evidence to prove an increase in the frequency of malformations or other harmful effects to the fetus. Animal studies show no evidence of an increased occurrence of fetal damage.

✔ **Category B2:** Drugs have been taken by only a limited number of pregnant women and women of childbearing age with no evidence to prove an increase in the frequency of malformations or other harmful effects to the fetus. No adequate animal studies are available, but the data that are available show no evidence of an increased occurrence of fetal damage.

✔ **Category B3:** Drugs have been taken by only a limited number of pregnant women and women of childbearing age with no evidence to prove an increase in the frequency of malformations or other harmful effects to the fetus. Studies in animals have shown evidence of an increased occurrence of fetal damage, but the significance is considered uncertain in humans.

The risks are so great that pregnant women should never take these drugs. Oral contraceptives are Category X drugs.

Rating reflux drugs

Before reading this section, check out Chapter 10, which is jam-packed with specific information about the various drugs used to treat heartburn/reflux. Then come right back.

Still here? Okay. I provide a scintillating explanation in the following short list and then sum up the info in a more expansive — and very specific — table (with brand names) in Table 17-1.

✔ **Over-the-counter (OTC) antacids** such as aluminum hydroxide, calcium carbonate, magnesium hydroxide, and sodium bicarbonate relieve heartburn simply by neutralizing the acid that backs up from your stomach into your esophagus. The virtue of this simplicity is that all these products are Category A drugs. They don't cross the placenta; they don't injure the fetus.

✔ **H2 blockers** cimetidine (Tagamet), famotidine (Pepcid), and ranitidine (Zantac) are more proactive, relieving reflux by reducing your stomach's natural secretion of acid. These drugs do cross the placenta, but animal studies show no evidence of fetal injury. Furthermore, no reports suggest any injury to human fetuses.

Better yet, when Canada's Motherisk Program compared 230 women with heartburn and 178 controls, the data showed no increase in fetal malfunctions among women using H2 blockers during the *first trimester* (first three months of pregnancy). They didn't find any differences later in pregnancy but still suggested more studies need to evaluate the second and third trimesters.

✔ The **proton pump inhibitor** omeprazole (Prilosec) also reduces the secretion of stomach juices and also crosses the placenta. But as of March 1997, Motherisk showed no difference in fetal outcomes between 59 pregnant women who had taken omeprazole and 178 controls (women who didn't take the drug).

Nonetheless, given the fact that many more women have taken the H2 blockers than have taken proton pump inhibitors, some experts, including the medical journal *Canadian Family Physician,* suggest that the H2 blockers may be the current drug of choice for pregnant women with heartburn/reflux.

Table 17-1	Comparing Reflux Remedies	
Medicine	*Brand Name*	*Pregnancy Classification*
OTC Antacids		
Aluminum compounds, calcium carbonate, magnesium compounds, sodium bicarbonate	Various	A
H2 Blockers		
Cimetidine	Tagamet Tagamet HB200* Enlon**	B(1)
Famotidine	Pepcid Pepcid AC* Acid Control**	B(1)
Nizatidine	Axid AR	B(1)(2)
Ranitidine	Zantac Zantac 75* Zantac C**	B(1)

(continued)

Table 17-1 *(continued)*

Medicine	Brand Name	Pregnancy Classification
Proton Pump Inhibitors		
Esomeprazole	Nexium	B(3)
Lansoprazole	Prevacid	B
Omeprazole	Prilosec Prilosec OTC* Losec**	C(1)(3)
Pantoprazole	Protonix	B
Rabeprazole	Aciphex	B

*Nonprescription product.
** Brand name in Canada.
(1) No adequate human studies available
(2) Drug produced abortions in pregnant rabbits.
(3) In doses up to 69 times the normal human dose, drug caused increase in fetal deaths in rats and rabbits. There have been some reports of congenital birth defects in babies born to women who used this drug while pregnant.
Sources: Rybacki, James, J. The Essential Guide to Prescription Drugs 2003 *(New York: Harper Resources, 2003); manufacturers' Web sites for specific drugs*

Filling in the (prescription) blanks

The FDA's current rules for describing drug safety during pregnancy concentrate on how the drug affects the fetus. However, you also need to know how pregnancy changes (or doesn't change) a woman's response to specific medicines.

When you're pregnant, your body changes in important ways that may affect how you process medicines. For example,

- ✔ Drugs circulate through your blood vessels. An increase in blood volume may change the concentration of a drug in your body.

- ✔ Some drugs are excreted in urine. When you urinate more frequently, you may decrease the amount of medicine you retain.

To make sure that you're taking the right drugs in the right strengths, always check with your doctor before adding a medicine.

Becoming a research person

A *pregnancy registry* is a study that enrolls pregnant women who are using specific medicines, such as antiseizure drugs. A woman enrolls in a registry when she is pregnant and taking the medicine. When her baby is born, the registry can compare the baby's health with that of infants born to women not taking this particular medicine.

The FDA Office of Women's Health (www.fda.gov/womens) keeps a list of pregnancy registries. To enroll in one, you must contact the people running the study who will tell you whether you can enroll yourself or need a recommendation from your doctor or pharmacist.

If you're accepted, the registry staff will probably want to interview you while you're pregnant and after you deliver the baby. Naturally, any information collected during these interviews is confidential. When the study is finished, reports of the results will be available to you. What is your reward? You get the satisfaction of having contributed to the effort to make drugs safer during pregnancy. You can find information about joining a pregnancy registry by

- ✔ Visiting the Web site of the Food and Drug Administration at www.fda.gov and typing "pregnancy registries" in the search box

- ✔ Going directly to the FDA's Office of Women's Health site at www.fda.gov/womens and following the link to registries provided

Examining home remedies

Simple home remedies for heartburn such as low-fat foods and smaller meals generally work as well for women who are pregnant as they do for other people. As soon as you move into the sort-of-medical realm — herbs, herbal products, and bicarbonate of soda (baking soda) are good examples — you should seek your doctor's advice and consent. ***Remember:*** Your aim is to protect your developing fetus while relieving that — burp! — unpleasant heartburn. Who better than your doctor to tell you how to accomplish your goal?

De-Linking Your Lifestyle from Your Reflux

When you're pregnant — just as when you're not — what you eat, how you sleep, what you wear, and how you exercise may play an important role in determining whether you end up with reflux.

Eating in comfort

A few simple changes in your menu and your meal schedule can go a long way toward helping to relieve pregnancy-related heartburn. You should

- ✔ **Avoid high-fat or greasy foods.** They loosen your LES and let food back into your esophagus.

- ✔ **Avoid very spicy foods.** Ditto on the loosening LES thing.

- ✔ **Cut way back on coffee.** The oil in coffee beans is a known heartburn trigger. If you must have caffeine, try tea; it has no oils and may be less upsetting.

- ✔ **Eat smaller meals, especially at dinner.** Your stomach can empty relatively quickly.

- ✔ **Limit consumption of carbonated beverages.** They make you burp which — surprise! — opens the LES.

- ✔ **Pass up bedtime snacks.** Why? The explanation is in the very next section.

For more on which foods and beverages trigger heartburn, check out Chapter 6.

Sleeping tight

Healthy women who aren't pregnant usually are awake during the day and sleeping through the night, but lugging around an extra 25 pounds or more can make a pregnant woman exhausted. Pregnant women are usually tired enough to slip in a couple of naps during the day. Maybe even tired enough to lie down right after eating, which isn't good.

As you can see in Chapter 14, climbing into bed right after eating isn't good behavior for people with reflux. And lying flat on your back, the easiest position to fall into late in pregnancy (wouldn't you know it?), flattens the digestive "tube" and makes it easier for acidic stomach contents to slide back into the esophagus.

You may reduce the incidence of this kind of reflux if you

- ✔ Nap sitting up in a comfortable chair

- ✔ Wait at least three hours after eating before lying down for the night, which is why bedtime snacks are a no-no

Twenty-three ways to say "I'm having a baby!"

Why has it been so hard for the human race to utter the simple word *pregnant?*

Yes, most people know that in order to get pregnant you have to take part in activities regarded as risqué by earlier generations who seem to have spent more energy making up euphemisms than it would take to raise a kid to college age.

But does that justify the lengths to which people have gone to avoid saying *p-r-e-g-n-a-n-t?*

Consider the Victorians. These delicate folk with a rigid sense of propriety called pregnant women *abundant, anticipating, expectant,* or *expecting.*

Members of the upper class who knew how to crook a pinky finger while lifting a cup of tea chose *enceinte* — plain French for (horrors!) pregnant.

For Classicists, the language of the Bible provided such fulsome terms as *with child, large with child,* or the prettily musical *childing.*

Plain folk, on the other hand, spoke plainly: Women were *gone, in an interesting condition,* or *in the family way.*

Naturally, the scientists chose science-speak: *gestating, gravid,* or *parturient.*

The Brits and the Irish showed their winning way with slang with *preggers,* not to mention the more-than-slightly gross *up the duff* (or *poke* or *pole* or *spout*).

Not to be outdone, the Americans put forth their own fairly gross *banged up* and *knocked up,* and then redeemed themselves with the homier Mom-and-apple-pie *bun in the oven.*

But who's kidding whom?

None of these substitutes comes within a mile of matching the joyous exuberance of *Honey! Guess what!*

Another way to reduce reflux while sleeping is to lie on your left side. Chapter 14 has the diagram showing why this helps, but the simple explanation is that

- ✔ Your stomach is on your left side.
- ✔ If you lie on the left, your stomach is lower than your esophagus.
- ✔ Your stomach contents are less likely to flow uphill, back into your esophagus.

Exercising caution

As a normal rule, just bending over can trigger reflux for some sensitive souls. Ditto for really bouncy exercises.

This goes double for pregnant women. As your pregnancy progresses, the sensible course is to stick to reasonable exercise such as mild stretching or a (relatively) brisk walk that keeps you upright while working your muscles as Chapter 14 explains.

Fashioning an alternative

Pregnant? Don't ignore your expanding waistline. Yes, you may want to fit into "regular" clothes for as long as possible. But clothes that are tight around the middle increase the risk of reflux. What else is there to say? Loosen up!

Chapter 18

Finding Heartburn in Infants and Children

*E*very so often — like right now — the author of a *For Dummies* book tells readers, "Hey, this chapter may not be for you." If your life is mostly children-free, you can flip past this chapter as long as you get the important message: Reflux is no respecter of age.

On the other hand, if you're a parent, grandparent, sister, brother, aunt, uncle, cousin, teacher, or babysitter who frequently spends time with one or more very young children, don't skip this chapter because it spells out which babies, infants, and young children are most at risk of reflux, shows you a list of symptoms that spell infant reflux, and dishes up tips on how to turn a crying baby into a bouncing bundle of joy.

Naming What's Making Your Child Cry

Once upon a time, pediatricians and parents thought heartburn and reflux were strictly for adults. Doctors thought babies who spit up all the time or cried all night had the undefined but common affliction called *colic.* Parents who stayed up all night with their children had sleep deprivation — but that's a subject for *Sleep Disorders For Dummies,* by Patricia B. Smith and Dr. Max Hirshkowitz (Wiley). Time flies.

Today, many doctors use the word *colicky* to describe an infant who cries about three hours a day. Some doctors simply translate colicky as "just plain irritable" or even label it a "term without a medical definition." What's happened? Modern medicine. Savvy pediatricians now consider the possibility of reflux when determining what's going on with babies who cry a lot, spit up, stay up, and don't seem to enjoy eating as much as most children.

A slew of up-to-the-minute research reports in prestigious medical journals supports the need to take a hard look at reflux in infants. One such journal, *Archives of Pediatrics & Adolescent Medicine* (`http://archpedi.ama-assn.org`), recently told its audience of baby docs that reflux is a "common disease of infancy" that affects up to 18 percent — about one in five — of otherwise healthy infants.

Identifying children at risk

Are you wondering if your own son or daughter or niece or nephew has reflux? Which children are most at risk for reflux? First, turn to Chapter 1 for a quick explanation of what reflux is. Basically, the lower esophageal sphincter (LES) is a trapdoor between the esophagus and stomach. If it fails to close tight, it can allow acidic stomach contents to flow back into the esophagus. Then fast forward to . . . right here.

As a general rule, the children who are most at risk are those with a medical condition that makes it difficult for them to breathe easily, to swallow food, or to maintain normal air pressure in the throat that holds the LES closed.

This list of children at risk of reflux includes those with

- **Chronic respiratory disease:** For example, children with cystic fibrosis or asthma are at greater risk.

- **Upper respiratory infection:** A cold, for example.

   Note: Although reflux may cause ear pain, no existing evidence proves a link between reflux and *otitis media,* a common ear infection in young children.

- **Frequent hiccups:** Hiccups increase pressure in the abdomen, which may cause acid to be refluxed back up into the esophagus.

- **Throat injuries:** Throat injuries may occur in infants due to respirators or breathing tubes used to help a premature infant breathe.

- **Structural irregularities:** Irregularities such as a *hiatal hernia,* a bit of the stomach that pushes up through a gap in the *diaphragm* (the muscular membrane that divides the chest from the abdomen) and into the chest (see Chapter 4 for more info).

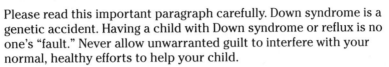

✔ **Food allergies or sensitivities:** Allergies and/or sensitivity reactions to foods may cause coughing or swelling of tissues that make it more difficult for a child to swallow.

✔ **Down syndrome:** This condition may weaken muscles or interfere with nerve impulses that keep the LES closed.

Please read this important paragraph carefully. Down syndrome is a genetic accident. Having a child with Down syndrome or reflux is no one's "fault." Never allow unwarranted guilt to interfere with your normal, healthy efforts to help your child.

✔ **Parents who suffer from reflux:** The tendency to reflux seems to run in families. If you have heartburn/reflux, keep an eye open because your pride and joy may have it, too. (Check out Chapter 4 for more on the family link associated with reflux.)

In fact, in 2000, the *Journal of the American Medical Association* published a report of five families with more than one child with reflux in which researchers suggested they may have located the "GERD gene" on chromosome 13. However, other researchers say more research is needed. Stay tuned.

Looking for signs of infant reflux

If you've ever held a baby, you know that babies spit up several times a day. As long as the spitting baby is smiling (a situation doctors characterize with the oh-so-technical term as a *happy spitter*) and you don't notice any other obvious medical problems, such as weight loss or tears at mealtime, then you don't have to worry. Childcare gurus often say that no kid goes off to kindergarten in diapers, and more than nine out of ten happy spitters outgrow the habit by their first birthday.

However, you're right to be concerned by frequent spitting up if

✔ Your baby doesn't gain weight.

✔ Your baby hiccups a lot.

✔ Your baby seems hungry but after one swallow refuses to continue nursing.

✔ Your baby is irritable or cries a lot for no obvious reason.

✔ Your baby is hoarse or has a persistent cough.

✔ Your baby has frequent choking episodes.

✔ Your baby has chronic nasal congestion caused by inhaling tiny food particles from her throat.

✔ Your baby has frequent bad breath.

Each of these signs suggests the possibility of reflux.

In addition, an observant parent may notice baby body language that shouts: Hey! I'm not happy here! For example, if your baby turns his head away from bottle or breast, becomes rigid, arches his back, or cries while feeding, he may be sending you a message. Figure 18-1 illustrates body language suggesting reflux.

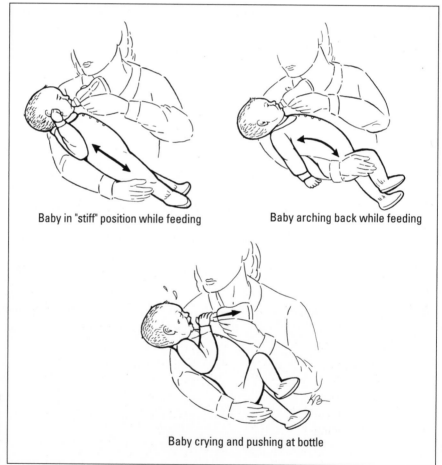

Baby in "stiff" position while feeding

Baby arching back while feeding

Baby crying and pushing at bottle

Figure 18-1:
Baby body
language.

Tracking reflux in toddlers

Unlike infants, toddlers and preschool children can talk. Maybe they don't recite the entire Gettysburg Address every morning before — or even after — breakfast, but they're capable of simple phrases such as "it hurts."

You may suspect reflux in your toddler when

- ✔ Your 2-year-old says it hurts to eat.
- ✔ Your 18-month-old wakes up in tears frequently during the night.
- ✔ Your child's asthma is worse at night.

These warning signs tell Dr. Mom or Dr. Dad to call Dr. Doctor the pediatrician or family physician for a professional checkup.

Diagnosing Reflux in Children

Gastroenterologists (the doctors who specialize in your digestive tract) have created several tests for diagnosing reflux in adults. After checking out Chapter 9, you can understand why doctors consider these tests stressful for grownups and practically impossible for infants and toddlers. As children grow older, some tests become useful.

To avoid unnecessary testing stress for an infant or toddler, your pediatrician is likely to make her first diagnosis of reflux via a combination of your reports of your child's symptoms and her own keen powers of observation.

If the result comes up reflux, your doctor may seek confirmation by referring your child to a pediatric gastroenterologist trained to

- ✔ Order a *scintigraphy,* a computerized scan of your child's abdomen to see how long it takes for food to pass out of the stomach. (The longer the food stays in the stomach, the higher the risk of reflux.)

- ✔ Prescribe an *upper GI series,* a radiological picture of the throat and stomach (the upper part of the gastrointestinal tract) after your child drinks a liquid that shows up on the film, outlining any defects or deformities.

- ✔ Insert a very small tube to measure acid levels in your child's throat, a guide to reflux of stomach contents.

- ✔ Perform *endoscopy,* a procedure during which your child is sedated so the doctor may insert a viewing tube into the infant's mouth and down through his throat to examine the esophagus, stomach, and intestines to check for reflux-related tissue damage.

Baby, you're the best

While you take some time to digest this fairly scary information, how about a movie break? The table below lists movies with *baby* in the title. Can you match the movie with the movie stars? Yes, the baby in one of these movies is actually a leopard. In a second, he's a dinosaur. In a third, a gangster. But, hey, every kid's special to its mom.

Movie Title (Year)	Movie Star(s)
1. Three Men and a Baby (1987)	a. Sean Young
2. Bringing Up Baby (1938)	b. Mickey Rooney
3. Baby Boom (1987)	c. Kevin Bacon
4. Baby Face (1933)	d. Tom Selleck
5. Baby Doll (1956)	e. Diane Keaton
6. The Babysitter (1995)	f. Carroll Baker
7. Baby . . . Secret of the Lost Legend (1985)	g. Katharine Hepburn, Cary Grant
8. She's Having a Baby (1988)	h. Barbara Stanwyck
9. Baby, the Rain Must Fall (1965)	i. John Mills
10. Baby Face Nelson (1957)	j. Lee Remick
11. The Baby and the Battleship (1956)	k. Shirley Temple
12. Baby Take a Bow (1934)	l. Alicia Silverstone

Answers: 1. d; 2. g; 3. e; 4. h; 5. f; 6. l; 7. a; 8. c; 9. j; 10. b; 11. i; 12. k

Treating Children with Reflux

After your doctor actually diagnoses your child's reflux, he must work out a treatment plan, following the North American Society of Pediatric Gastroenterology, Hematology, and Nutrition (NASPGHAN) guidelines.

In 2001, based on the growing evidence of reflux in children, NASPGHAN created a committee to draw up guidelines for treating youngsters with reflux.

Are you the intensely curious sort? If so, you can read the whole 20-plus-page report at the NASPGHAN Web site, `www.naspghan.org`. On the home page, click *Medical Professionals.* Choose the *Position Papers* link and then read the *Guidelines for the Evaluation and Treatment of Gastroesophageal Reflux in Infants and Children.*

The report contains a lot of medical jargon and is very repetitive. If your eyes begin to glaze around the second page, save it for another day.

Feeding well, feeling better

Reflux is a digestive problem, so the first line of defense is a well-tuned diet and feeding plan that eliminates reflux triggers. This advice sounds simple, but as you read the next several paragraphs, you may find a liberal sprinkling of the words *some* and *may.* Why? Because currently the data on infant reflux is in its infancy.

In other words, many expert suggestions are just that, suggestions rather than hard-and-fast rules.

Avoiding allergens

May, some, and *suggest* are very important words in science writing. These words flag an iffy subject such as the possibility of a link between allergenic foods and childhood reflux.

For example, *some* studies *suggest* that *some* babies who are sensitive to cow's milk *may* develop reflux when given cow's milk formulas. For children eating solid food, the list of potential allergens expands to include citrus fruit, including tomatoes. The theory is that an allergic reaction *may* loosen the LES and trigger reflux.

If a food allergen is to blame for your infant's discomfort, then switching to breastfeeding *may* solve the problem. Despite the growing popularity of breast-feeding, no evidence exists to prove that breastfed babies are less likely than bottle-fed babies to have reflux.

However, to test the allergen-equals-reflux proposition and possibly ease your baby's discomfort, your doctor may sensibly suggest a two-week elimination diet to find out which food may be the culprit.

A *two-week elimination diet* starts with a menu that's free of virtually all poten-tially allergenic foods. Then foods are added back one at a time. For example, eggs one day, milk the next, and so on. After each food is added, you watch for a reaction. If none occurs, you cross that food off the Troublesome List, and go on to the next.

If you're breastfeeding, what you eat ends up in your milk, so the elimination diet is for you, too. If you have reflux and are taking medication, check with your doctor to see if you should breastfeed. For more information on the reproductive effects of antireflux meds, check out Chapter 10.

Dishing up smaller meals

Sometimes, just giving your child smaller, more frequent feedings alleviates reflux. My, what an easy remedy, right?

Of course, you want to make sure that your child gets all the necessary nutrients, so you don't cut down the total amount of food you serve each day, just reduce the portion size and serve more frequent meals so your child isn't hungry. Read all about the antireflux benefits of smaller portions and more-frequent meals in Chapter 6.

Thickening the formula

This recommendation for infants is another slightly iffy one. NASPGHAN says the good news is that thickened formulas — milk plus a cereal — reduces the incidence of spitting up. The so-so news is that no studies exist to show that thickened formulas reduce the reflux.

Additionally, consider the following points when thickening your baby's food:

✔ Consider using rice to thicken the formula or pumped breast milk. Rice is less likely than other grains to set allergy bells ringing. But of course check with your doctor to be sure.

✔ Know that thickened formulas may increase a baby's coughing while feeding.

✔ If the thickened milk stays longer in the stomach, it may actually be *more* likely to slip back through the LES. In other words, a thickened formula may make your infant more comfortable — or maybe not.

Serving a pacifier for dessert

In Chapter 7, I share how chewing gum can be a weapon in the war against reflux for adults. Chewing increases the production of *saliva,* a natural antacid that helps neutralizes fiery reflux in the esophagus.

The infant equivalent of chewing gum may be a pacifier. Sucking on this substitute breast not only increases the secretion of saliva but also stimulates *peristalsis,* the natural contractions of the intestinal tract that move food along, out of the stomach and down through the body. Alas, right now no studies are available to prove the point. However, less food sitting in the tummy means less risk of reflux.

Moving on to preschool

Like some adults, some preschool children may react badly to high-fat foods, spicy foods, soft drinks, and chocolate (which has caffeine), all of which are known to loosen the LES. Eliminating these foods from your child's diet may alleviate his reflux (see Chapter 6 for more on these red-flag foods).

Picking a perfect position

Possession, they say, is nine-tenths of the law. Position can be equally important to helping your child enjoy her meals, nap nicely during the day, and sleep tight at night.

Positioning your baby for a happy feeding

Adults with reflux usually know from unhappy experience that lying down while eating or right afterwards allows acidic stomach contents to slide back into the esophagus. The same is true for nursing infants.

So, place your infant in a sort of upright position while feeding and keep her sort of upright for a while after the feeding is done. I say "sort of" because no infant is actually going to sit up straight at the dinner table. The reflux researchers' proposal is that you hold or position your baby at a 45- to 60-degree angle while feeding him. If you haven't majored in geometry, check out Figure 18-2. After he's eaten, keep him "sort of" upright in a baby sling or chair.

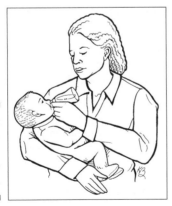

Figure 18-2:
Feeding baby at a 45-degree angle.

Lying down for a good night's sleep

An older child, like adults, may cut his risk of nighttime GERD by sleeping on his left side, a position that puts the stomach below the throat, thus reducing the back-flow of acid (see Chapter 14).

Some studies suggest a similar effect for babies, and the NASPGHAN guidelines note that infant reflux may be as much as three times more common among babies who sleep on their backs than among those babies who sleep on their tummies.

If life were simple, the lesson would be clear: To avoid nighttime infant reflux, put babies to sleep on their left side or on their stomach. Alas, life is never, ever simple. Although sleeping face down is fine for older children, alert parents know that infants in this position are at higher risk of sudden infant death syndrome (SIDS). Because the risk of SIDS in babies up to 12 months old far outweighs the benefits of reducing reflux, the American Academy of Pediatrics (AAP) says infants may lie on their tummies while awake but make sure they always sleep on their backs. Even during waking hours, the AAP says never, ever place an infant face down on soft bedding, which increases the risk of SIDS.

Medicating childhood reflux

The medical treatment for reflux in infants and children is pretty much the same as that for Mom and Dad: Use medicines to reduce or neutralize stomach acid and surgery to repair the LES.

Finding a friend

When your child is sick, your family and friends may offer sincere sympathy and support, but nothing beats the company of someone who knows exactly what you're experiencing. In other words, talk to the parent of a child with reflux or a group of parents of children with reflux.

The Pediatric/Adolescent Gastroesophageal Reflux Association (PAGER) is a nonprofit membership organization founded by GERD parents to provide information and support to others in the same situation. The group includes medical explanations for people without medical degrees, a forum where parents can exchange information, news about ongoing clinical studies (including one on the genetic basis for reflux), and best of all, volunteers who can answer your questions online or over the phone. Connect with PAGER at www.reflux.org or 866-KID-GERD or 301-601-9541.

Another support source is La Leche League International, the breastfeeding advocacy organization. Although simply switching from bottles to breast or vice versa isn't a cure for reflux, La Leche is a fountainhead of useful feeding tips. Click onto the home page at www.lalecheleague.org/, type "reflux" in the search bar, and then scroll down a list of helpful links.

Choosing children's medicines

Chapter 10 is a complete guide to the variety of prescription drugs and over-the-counter (OTC) products used to relieve heartburn/reflux in adults. Some studies show that these medicines are safe and effective for children and infants, but the data are — to put it mildly — scanty.

The following list from the NASPGHAN guidelines demonstrates the limited nature of infant studies. By the time you read this, more information may be available. But the main rule still pertains: Never, ever give your infant or young child an antacid or heartburn medicine without your pediatrician's advice and consent. (Come to think of it, that rule applies for any condition.)

- A few small studies suggest that omeprazole (brand name Prilosec) reduces the acidity of reflux that reaches an infant's esophagus and may be helpful in treating respiratory problems in babies resulting from reflux.

- One study of 32 infants showed cimetidine (Tagamet) helped heal esophageal tissue damaged by reflux. One study of 24 infants showed similar results with nizatidine (Axid). No similar research has studied ranitidine (Zantac) or famotidine (Pepcid).

- OTC antacids, such as magnesium hydroxide plus aluminum hydroxide (Maalox Plus, Mylanta, and so on), appear to be effective, but antacids containing aluminum may raise blood levels of aluminum, thus increasing the risk of bone damage, anemia, and nerve damage in infants and young children.

No researchers seem to have conducted infant studies of single-ingredient antacids made with either calcium carbonate (Tums) or magnesium hydroxide.

Selecting surgery

When medicine doesn't relieve a child's reflux, surgery to repair a malfunctioning LES may be an option. See Chapter 12 for the procedures used to treat GERD. Consult with your doctor because the surgery may be more difficult for a small baby than for a full-grown adult.

Chapter 19

Taking Aim at Senior Heartburn

. . . .

In This Chapter

▶ Facing heartburn as you grow older (and better)

▶ Listing signs of reflux in older folks

▶ Identifying heartburn in seniors

▶ Taking care of senior heartburn

. . . .

*H*eartburn is so common among senior citizens that many people accept it as another normal consequence of aging. However, as common as heartburn may be, it's never normal. So don't feel that you can — or should — sit back and simply accept the pain.

Doctors can treat heartburn and reflux among the older set as effectively as they take care of it in young whippersnappers (a neat term which — sadly — seems to have gone the way of the dinosaurs and the Model T).

Although physical changes in an aging body may affect how doctors diagnose and treat heartburn, when a sensible patient and a patient doctor get together, there's no stopping them: Diagnosing and treating heartburn can become relatively simple to accomplish. As always, the goal is an active, pain-free life. At any age!

Aging into Heartburn

How can you tell if you're getting older? Let me count the ways:

✔ At the cosmetic counter, you pass up the oil-free products and head for the ones marked "dry skin."

✔ You discover gray hair — and a newfound interest in hair-coloring products.

✔ You don't roll your eyes anymore when others say stuff like, "It's going to rain today; I can feel it in my bones" — because you can too!

✔ You aren't eating more, but you're putting on pounds.

✔ After you stop laughing, the lines at the corner of your mouth are still there. After you frown, the lines in the middle of your forehead don't go away, either.

✔ Miniskirts and rock-hard abs are a memory; the new reality is spider veins and flab.

✔ When you dig into a simple meal of hot dogs and beans, or grilled cheese, or a chicken salad, or anything else — no matter what you eat — you end up with heartburn.

Rising risks

Reflux has no age requirements, but it does seem to favor senior citizens. In fact, as the golden years approach, the risk of reflux rises sharply. Consider the following statistics, according to the National Institutes of Health (NIH) and the National Heartburn Alliance (NHBA):

✔ More than half of the Americans with reflux problems are age 45 to 65.

✔ More than 30 percent of women older than 65 have frequent heartburn.

And would you believe that more than half of the people older than 55 who have heartburn think that it's all their fault because they ate the wrong food or because they had one cocktail before dinner. Of course, they're wrong. The fault isn't in yourself, but in your body.

Soaring severity

Older patients with reflux are also likely to experience more complications than younger patients with reflux, and their complications are likely to be more severe.

A recent report in the *American Journal of Gastroenterology* estimated that as many as one in four reflux sufferers older than 60 had developed *Barrett's esophagus,* the tissue damage linked to an increased risk of esophageal cancer. Among those sufferers younger than 60, the incidence was about one in seven. (For more Barrett's info and stats, turn back to Chapter 3.)

Older people with reflux are also more likely to have damaged teeth. Dental enamel is extraordinarily strong, but it can't withstand constant exposure to a backwash of acid stomach liquids.

Medical school students are often told to "look for horses, not zebras," a clever way of saying "look for the simplest explanation first." In this case, the "horse" is almost certainly the obvious fact that older people with reflux have had their problem for a longer period of time, which means they also had longer exposure to the damaging effects of acid reflux, such as continued irritation to the esophagus (leading to Barrett's) or that acidic assault on the teeth.

Identifying the Risk Factors in Older Folk

Dry skin, gray hair, and permanent smile lines are some of the relatively benign changes that come naturally with the years. Others changes, such as osteoporosis, are more serious. And some changes increase the risk of reflux.

Losing muscle power

As you age, you experience a gradual loss of muscle strength, and your digestive tract is comprised of a number of muscles. When your digestive muscles get flabby, you get heartburn.

Every day, your body builds new cells and tissues to replace those cells lost in the ordinary course of life. Your body utilizes the nutrients from your well-balanced diet to generate new cells and body tissues. (Check out my book *Nutrition For Dummies,* published by Wiley, for tips on creating a well-balanced diet.)

To make muscles, you need protein, the important nutrient your body uses to synthesize new proteins, such as *hemoglobin* (the protein in red blood cells that carries oxygen to all your tissues), and the protein-rich tissue called muscle. But an older body synthesizes proteins less efficiently, and older people build less new muscle tissue.

As you grow older, your digestive muscles, like all your body's muscles, tend to relax and lose some strength. Working out can help counteract the loss of power in your skeletal muscles — arms, legs, abs, and so on — but no one has yet invented effective exercises for digestive muscles.

As Chapter 2 explains, your digestive tract is ringed with strong muscles that contract in waves called *peristalsis* that push food to your esophagus, and then down through a circular gateway called the lower esophageal sphincter (LES) into your stomach. After the food reaches your stomach, the LES closes to keep food and stomach acid from moving back into your esophagus. Occasionally, the LES doesn't close tight or opens by mistake, allowing acidic stomach contents to flow back. This phenomenon is reflux. The reflux produces the burning sensation called heartburn.

So how do aging muscles increase the risk of reflux? The three following possibilities emerge.

✔ A weakened LES increases the chances that food and stomach acid will flow back into your esophagus.

✔ When acidic stomach contents slosh back past the LES into your esophagus, the esophageal muscles are designed to contract strongly enough to push the burning liquids back down where they belong. But an older person's esophageal muscles may contract less vigorously. Result? Heartburn.

✔ The muscles where the esophagus enters the stomach may gap, and a *hiatal hernia* — a small part of your stomach pushing up through the gap into your chest cavity — may occur. This pressure also weakens the LES. Result? More heartburn.

Losing gland power

When you're talking heartburn, the glands that matter are the salivary glands. As Figure 19-1 shows, you have three major pairs of salivary glands, each pair named for its location in your body.

Facing the fat

As you grow older, you make less muscle tissue, but your fat factory perks along at normal speed, so the amount of fatty (*adipose*) tissue in your body stays the same or — horrors! — increases. The result? You may look like your muscles are "turning to fat" when in fact you're actually losing muscle tissue while holding (or building) fatty tissue.

Older women notice this effect more than older men because, by nature, men have more muscle mass than women.

Generally,

✔ The average adult female body has proportionately more fatty tissue than the average male body.

✔ The average adult male body has proportionately more muscle tissue than the average female body.

As a result, in old age, a woman has less muscle to lose, so any loss at all is clearly noticeable.

The following list shows the derivation of the names for the salivary glands, a bonus for those of you who share my fascination with etymology.

✔ The *parotid salivary glands,* the largest of the three pairs, are located at the angle of your jaw, under your ears (from the Greek *para* for *around,* *-ot* for *ear*).

✔ The *submandibular salivary glands* are located under your jaw (from the Latin, *mando* for *jaw*).

✔ The *sublingual salivary glands* are located on the floor of your mouth under your tongue (from the Latin *lingua* for *tongue*).

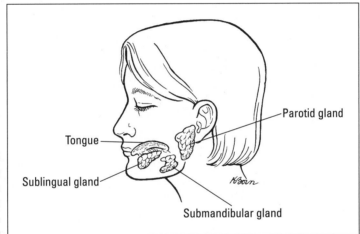

Tongue

Parotid gland

Sublingual gland

Submandibular gland

Figure 19-1: Getting in touch with your glands.

The primary function of these three pairs of salivary glands is to secrete saliva, a mineral-rich liquid that, among other things

✔ Hardens your teeth

✔ Moistens and protects your tongue and the lining of your mouth

✔ Moistens food so you can swallow it easily

Salivary glands play an important role in the defense against heartburn and reflux because saliva also

✔ Neutralizes acid reflux in your esophagus (for more details, check out Chapter 2)

✔ Flows down your esophagus to push reflux back into your stomach (again, the details are in Chapter 2)

When aging salivary glands produce less saliva, acid reflux is likely to linger longer in the esophagus and to burn stronger.

Multiplying meds

Chronic health problems such as arthritis and high blood pressure become more common as the years go by; even healthy senior citizens are likely to be taking several medicines — both prescription drugs and over-the-counter (OTC) products — every day.

As a smart medical consumer, you know that all meds come with baggage: the risk of adverse side effects and interactions. Multiply the risks by two, three, four, or more different medicines a day, and side effects, including heartburn, become a fact of life.

One example of meds commonly taken by many older folks that cause gastric problems is *nonsteroidal anti-inflammatory drugs* (NSAIDs) such as ibuprofen. NSAIDs are in the first line of defense against arthritis. Unfortunately, NSAIDs are also high on the list of drugs that upset the stomach.

For a list of other medicines that may causes heartburn in people of any age, turn to Chapter 11. Also check out "Prescribing relief" later in this chapter for a short list of drug interactions that may occur in older people taking antireflux drugs along with other common drugs. More reasons to show you why old age isn't for sissies.

Lying down

Being "bed bound" — unable to get up and about due to injury, illness, or the frailty of old age — can raise your risk of reflux-related heartburn. The main culprit is your being pretty much flat on your back, a position in which stomach contents are more likely to slosh back through the LES into your esophagus.

To minimize the problem and make you more comfortable, your doctor may recommend that your caregivers

✔ Raise the head of your bed, a technique I describe in Chapter 16 as a method for reducing the risk of nighttime reflux (reflux while you're sleeping)

✔ Help you sit up during meals

✔ Help you get out of bed during the day, if possible, so you can be upright for a while after meals

Diagnosing Heartburn in Older Patients

Because older patients generally have more medical problems than younger patients do, doctors sometimes have a difficult time separating out the symptoms to arrive at a reasonable diagnosis.

The primary symptom of esophageal reflux is the episodic pain that may wander up and down the chest. That symptom is good at imitating heart attack, which is why so many people with heartburn trundle themselves off to the emergency room. A careful doctor facing a patient past retirement age will likely decide to rule out the latter before diagnosing the former.

Another surprising fact is an age-related loss of sensitivity to specific sources of pain and/or discomfort. Several studies as recently as 2000 in the United States and Europe have shown that

- When gastrointestinal researchers inserted a balloon into the esophagus of volunteers and gradually filled the balloon with air, young subjects report discomfort when the balloon was only slightly inflated. Older subjects don't complain until later.

- When researchers drip a diluted acid solution into the esophagus, older volunteers tolerate the drip for longer periods of time before they feel pain.

You may think that not feeling pain is good, but the condition has drawbacks, especially for people with reflux. If you don't feel reflux pain, you don't complain. If you don't complain, your reflux won't be diagnosed. If your reflux isn't diagnosed, it won't be treated. If your reflux isn't treated, the damage to your esophagus continues. And that, ladies and gentlemen, is what may explain why older people often have more serious esophageal damage.

To rein in the damage, the American College of Gastroenterology's (ACG) guidelines for reflux disease suggests a number of "alarm symptoms" for people older than 65 to be aware of. If you experience any of these symptoms, see your doctor and let her perform appropriate diagnostics tests to get a handle on what's causing your symptoms. You can read more about diagnostic tests for reflux in Chapter 9.

- Pain when swallowing

- Esophageal bleeding

- Unintended loss of more than 5 percent of body weight

- Choking or trouble breathing

- Chest pain not linked to heart disease

Geri-who?

Geriatrics — from the Greek words *geras* (old age) and *iatrikos* (healing) — is the branch of medicine devoted to the care of older people. Specialists often add the prefix *geri-* or the adjective geriatric to their titles. For example, a geriatric physician is a primary care physician for senior citizens.

Speaking of which, what do you call someone older than you? Other than Mom and Dad, or Grandma or Grandpa. *Sexagenarian* (age 60–69), *septuagenarian* (age 70– 79), *octagenarian* (80– 89), *nonagenarian* (90–99), and *centarian* (older than 100) are accurate but awkward. *Aged* and

elderly are dignified, but dull. *Gray* and *grizzled* are messy. *Gone to seed, past one's prime,* and *on the shelf* sound like moldy cheese. *Ancient* and *hoary* are classic but rare. *Senior citizen* and *golden ager* are too cute for words. *Geezer* is demeaning; so are *granny, pop, old gal,* and *old fella. Seasoned* and *mature* are okay, but not great.

In a society that finds great words for old wines, why can't anyone do better? Who, as one American company once nicely put it, "aren't getting older; they're getting better." Suggestions, anyone?

Treating Senior Heartburn

The treatments for older people with heartburn are basically the same as those for younger people — lifestyle, medicine, and surgery. The distinction, as always, lies in the details.

Modifying your lifestyle

You may grow older, but the lifestyle advice on reflux remains the same. Integrate into your life the following steps to improve your health:

- Avoid foods that cause heartburn.
- Control your weight.
- Don't eat for three hours before going to bed.
- Don't smoke.
- Eat smaller meals.
- Tailor your exercise regimen to your reflux sensitivity.

Most importantly, check with your doctor before you make any drastic lifestyle changes. He can assist you with certain foods to avoid and what exercises are appropriate for you.

Following these rules may alleviate your heartburn, but following these rules may feel restrictive. Life is full of choices. Making them is what life is all about — regardless of your age.

Prescribing relief

Pretend you're a doctor who's just diagnosed reflux in an older person. What's your next step? Simple, you say. You tell the person to try an ordinary OTC antacid and see if that helps.

Suppose I tell you that plain old antacids such as calcium carbonate can interfere with the absorption of other drugs, or that they can cause constipation, a major complaint among the older set. True, you say, but magnesium antacids aren't constipating, so you may prescribe them instead for patients who complain of constipation.

Good for you. You've found a rational alternative. But you've also discovered that some older people may have specific problems with common meds. They may also have trouble with common forms of those meds, thus requiring liquids rather than hard-to-swallow pills and tablets.

And with interactions, the difficulties multiply. The good news about the new, more effective antireflux medicines such as H2 blockers — cimetidine (Tagamet) — and proton pump inhibitors also known as PPIs — omeprazole (Prilosec) — is that they're safe for elderly patients. The bad news is that they, like the plain old antacids, interact with other drugs seniors are likely to be using. Table 19-1 lists some possible interactions.

Table 19-1	Aging Interactions
Medicine	*May Interact with Drugs for These Age-Related Conditions*
OTC Antacids	
Products containing sodium	Heart disease, high blood pressure
H2 Blockers	
Cimetidine (Tagamet)	Arthritis, depression, diabetes, heart disease, erectile dysfunction, prostate disease
Famotidine (Pepcid)	Arthritis, heart disease
Nizatidine (Axid)	Arthritis, heart disease
Ranitidine (Zantac)	Anxiety, arthritis, diabetes, heart disease

(continued)

Table 19-1 *(continued)*	
Medicine	*May Interact with Drugs for These Age-Related Conditions*
Proton Pump Inhibitors	
Esomeprazole (Nexium)	Anxiety, heart disease
Lansoprazole (Prevacid)	Liver disease
Omeprazole (Prilosec)	Anxiety, arthritis, heart disease
Pantoprazole (Protonex)	Not yet available
Rabeprazole (Actiphex)	Not yet available

Source: *Rybacki, James J.,* The Essential Guide to Prescription Drugs *(New York: Harper Collins, 2003); product package inserts (available 2003)*

Cutting options

As Chapter 12 explains, heartburn surgery is almost always an elective — rather than a required — procedure. In addition, it is the last resort, used only if medicines and lifestyle changes don't alleviate the burn.

Nonetheless, the introduction of minimally invasive surgery, or laparoscopic procedures, has reduced the trauma of many forms of surgery. Start with the fact that the laparoscopic technique permits the surgeon to operate via a much smaller incision and enables the surgeon to do the surgery more quickly, requiring less time under the anesthetic, and patients recover faster.

Today doctors now use laparoscopic techniques for reflux surgery (see Chapter 12). Older people — who may be poor surgical risks because of heart disease, poor circulation, high blood pressure, and respiratory difficulty — can benefit from laparoscopic techniques.

However, make sure your doctor thoroughly evaluates you to determine whether your risks of surgery outweigh the benefits and to see if you're a viable candidate. It's a pretty safe bet that a larger number of older people will flunk the test based on their general health, but some will pass. If ever there were a situation in which the decision must be made one person at a time, this is it.

Aging populations

Forget the Baby Boom. The wave of the future is the Geezer Geyser. Although life is still tragically too short in many nonindustrialized nations, with new medicines and improved living conditions people in the industrialized world are still alive — and still active — long past what used to be considered old age.

In 1900, the Centers for Disease Control (CDC) reported the life expectancy for men in the United States at 46.3 years and for women at 48.3. A century later, things sure have changed. According to population studies from the United Nations, the 65-year-old-and-up population is a growth market in the United States and seven major industrialized nations: Australia, Canada, France, Germany, Japan, New Zealand, and the United Kingdom.

Leading the way is Japan where the percentage of the population older than 65 will grow by more than 50 percent in the next two decades. By 2020, one of every four Japanese citizens will be older then 65. In Germany, France, and the United Kingdom, the 2020 ratio will be one in five. In Canada, Australia, New Zealand, and the United States, it will be one in six.

On average, just as in 1900, women still live longer than men do, a situation many attribute to genetics. Women have two X chromosomes (men have one X plus one Y), and geneticists say the double X combination is more protective.

The result is an increasingly female older population. A recent report from The Commonwealth Fund, an international think tank, says that although more boys than girls are born, by age 65 there are about nine men for every ten women. Fifteen years later, at age 80, the ratio is five men for every ten women. If you're a lady looking for a date or a guy just looking to survive, you don't want to know what happens by 100! By the way, Japan, which projects the largest increase in the number of old people, also has the greatest number of parents living with their children. Anyone want to draw a conclusion from that?

Where you live clearly affects your longevity. Check out the following table, which presents United Nations numbers on the percentage of total population age 65 and older.

Country	% 2000	% 2020 (estimate)	% Change
Australia	12.1	16.8	+39
Canada	12.8	18.2	+43
France	15.9	20.1	+26
Germany	16.4	21.6	+32
Japan	17.1	26.2	+54
New Zealand	11.6	15.6	+34
United Kingdom	16.0	19.8	+24
United States	12.5	16.6	+33

Part VI
The Part of Tens

The 5th Wave   By Rich Tennant

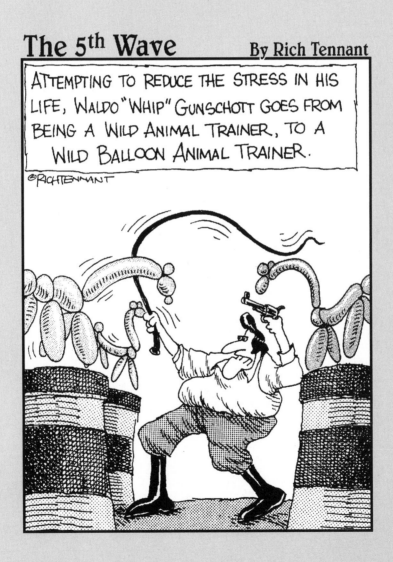

ATTEMPTING TO REDUCE THE STRESS IN HIS LIFE, WALDO "WHIP" GUNSCHOTT GOES FROM BEING A WILD ANIMAL TRAINER, TO A WILD BALLOON ANIMAL TRAINER.

In this part . . .

This is the one known as The Fun Part where you find a list of heartburn myths (and an explanation of why they're wrong), great Web sites for people with heartburn, and a list of common digestive disorders. Okay, so that last one doesn't sound like fun. But won't you be relieved to know what disorders you *don't* have? Yes, you will.

Chapter 20

Ten or So Heartburn and Reflux Myths

Myth-information is the enemy of good medicine, especially with conditions as common as heartburn and reflux. Like the common cold, common heartburn seems to inspire home remedies and old wives' tales.

For example, your friend's cousin's brother-in-law swears he cured his heartburn by sucking on peppermints after eating, and your brother's wife's mother relies on a soothing snifter of brandy after dinner.

But you may be surprised to hear that peppermint is actually one of the foods and flavorings that makes heartburn more likely. And Chapter 14 says that alcohol is usually a no-no for people with reflux.

Because I've just debunked these two heartburn myths, you don't find them in this chapter. But you can read about the real risk of heartburn-related cancer and the link (or lack thereof) between your weight and gender and your heartburn.

Finally, this chapter answers that burning question: What does heartburn have to do with your heart? That's the 12th myth in this list of ten, but I won't tell if you won't.

Heartburn Is Common, So It's Nothing to Worry About

Yes, the stats in Chapter 1 say that heartburn is common. *Webster's New World College Dictionary* defines *common* as "belonging or relating to the community at large." But who said that *common* means *nothing to worry about?*

The annoying pain in your middle is a real medical condition that, left untreated, may escalate into real medical trouble, such as the precancerous condition called Barrett's esophagus or even the Big C itself. The good news, of course, is that these consequences rarely develop, and you may prevent them by treating your heartburn with the respect (and medicine) it deserves.

In other words, got heartburn? Get relief. Now.

Heartburn and Reflux Inevitably Lead to Cancer

This statement, the opposite of the first myth in this chapter, is equally over the line. According to the *Journal of the American Medical Association,* heartburn is common, and esophageal cancer is rare.

University of North Carolina (Chapel Hill) medical researchers Nicholas Shaheen and David Ransohoff wanted to find out whether it makes sense to have everyone with heartburn and reflux tested for esophageal cancer. Crunching numbers on their handy-dandy calculators, they discovered that 10 million Americans age 50 and over have at least one incident of heartburn and reflux a week, but only 3,900 of these folks develop cancer of the esophagus.

In other words (or other numbers), there's a 0.039 percent risk that any one person with heartburn and reflux will develop cancer of the esophagus — roughly 4 in 10,000. Whew! (Consumer alert! For specific info on who does need to be tested for esophageal cancer, check out Chapter 3.)

Only Overweight People, Drinkers, and Chiliheads Get Heartburn and Reflux

Yes, being overweight, smoking, drinking, or eating spicy foods may light that familiar burning sensation. But no, being a skinny teetotaler on a bland diet doesn't guarantee protection from heartburn.

Alas, heartburn may strike people with no obvious triggers. Some people are just more susceptible than others due to factors like their lifestyle or their genes (heartburn does seem to run in families).

Sorry about that.

Smoking a Cigarette After Eating Prevents Heartburn

If this myth hadn't popped up on the National Institute of Diabetes and Digestive and Kidney Diseases (NIDDK) Web site (www.niddk.nih.gov), where it's handily debunked, I wouldn't have included it here.

Of course, smoking doesn't prevent heartburn. Although smoking relaxes many people, it also loosens the lower esophageal sphincter (LES), the opening from your stomach to your esophagus, thus increasing your risk of heartburn.

But you knew that, right? If not, read more about how smoking affects the LES in Chapter 14.

Heartburn Is an Inevitable Part of Growing Older

Like several other organs and body parts, your digestive system does slow down a bit as you grow older. That's why constipation plagues senior citizens . . . and so does heartburn. But heartburn and reflux are never inevitable. As your doctor is delighted to explain, you can ease the pain at any age. Moving on . . .

OTC Antacids Aren't Real Medicine

You don't need a doctor's prescription to buy over-the-counter (OTC) medicines, but like any product used to treat a medical condition, OTC meds deserve your respect.

When used with the advice of your physician or as directed on the package, OTC antacids are generally safe and effective. However, like any other medicines, these antacids may interact with other drugs or trigger unpleasant side effects.

For example, normal doses of calcium antacids can prevent your body from absorbing some antibiotics (such as the tetracyclines), and very large doses can cause constipation. OTC antacids containing magnesium, another acid neutralizer, may have just the opposite effect (diarrhea), and they are potentially hazardous for people with kidney disease.

Bottom line: A drug is a drug is a drug. Check out Chapter 10 for the full scoop on meds and heartburn.

Taking Prescription Heartburn and Reflux Drugs Makes Digesting Food More Difficult

In the natural course of human events, your stomach secretes hydrochloric acid (HCl), which works hand in hand with the protein compounds called *enzymes* to digest practically any food you can toss down your gullet. As a secondary benefit, HCl does a fine job of knocking off many potentially harmful bacteria that ride in on the food.

Many people worry that prescription drugs for heartburn or reflux reduce the amount of acid in their stomachs to the point that they won't be able to digest food properly. Although these prescription drugs do slow the natural HCl secretion, the stomach never completely stops secreting HCl. As a result, you always produce sufficient stomach acids to digest your foods.

Note: OTC antacids have no effect on acid secretion; they *neutralize* stomach acids, making them less irritating to your esophagus.

Having Nighttime Heartburn Means You Should Sleep Sitting Up

No, but you may be more comfortable sleeping on your left side. Your stomach is one section of a long tube that starts at your mouth and runs all the way down to the other end of your body. As the diagram of your innards in Chapter 2 shows, your stomach is positioned to the left of your esophagus. Stick a bookmark in the page and turn back to check out the picture.

Okay: Now with that fixed firmly in your mind, think about what happens if you lie flat on your back. The digestive "tube" flattens out so that liquid from your stomach can flow relatively easily back into your esophagus. If you lie on your right side, your stomach is higher than your esophagus, which means that stomach liquids may flow *down* into your throat. If that happens, the liquids have a really, really hard time flowing back *up* into your stomach.

But lie on your left side, and voila! The digestive tube is no longer flat, and the stomach is downhill from your esophagus. So acidic stomach contents are less likely to flow backwards into your throat.

By the way, this theory holds for any time you lie down: On a beach blanket, watching football on Monday night, swinging in a hammock — the left side is the right side.

Love Coffee? Got Heartburn? Switch to Decaf

Waste of time, guys, waste of time. The only difference between regular coffee and decaf is the presence (or absence) of caffeine, and caffeine isn't the ingredient that sets your stomach ablaze. The offending ingredients in coffee are the naturally occurring oils that give the coffee beans their flavor and *mouth-feel* — the way coffee feels in your mouth.

Can't face a caffeine-free morning? Try tea or *mate* (or *yerba mate*), the South American beverage made from the leaves and twigs of a tree that grows in Argentina, Paraguay, and Peru.

Mate may have as much caffeine per cup as coffee (about 100 mg), and tea has half as much. In *moderate* amounts, both tea and mate are less likely to cause heartburn. Of course, I don't need to point out that I set the word *moderate* in *italics* to emphasize that moderate means two or three cups a day, not 12. Really.

To Avoid Heartburn After Eating, Relax

Maybe not. As the National Heartburn Alliance (NHBA) notes, physical activity helps to keep the digestive system moving, which means that the stomach empties out, reducing the risk of it spitting its contents back up into your esophagus.

Of course, the NHBA means moderate (there's that word again!) exercise. No weight lifting. No 30-second sprints. Just a nice walk around a couple of blocks, or down the lane, or . . . well, whatever keeps you moving without jiggling your organs around so energetically that your stomach contents bounce up into your esophagus.

Having Heartburn during Pregnancy Means Giving Birth to a Hairy Baby

The first time I heard this myth, I nearly fell down laughing. After the second and third times, though, I thought I should put that in my list of ten myths about heartburn/reflux. So, no, heartburn isn't a predictor of hairy infants.

The question is, how did this myth become so widespread? When I checked out its origins, I discovered that it shows up all over the world. (Anyone who can tell me where this myth started gets a mention in a future edition of this book.)

Heartburn Is Connected to the Heart

No, no. A thousand times — no. You feel the pain in the middle of your chest, which makes most people think of the heart. That's how this condition got its name. The pros prefer to call the condition reflux or gastroesophageal reflux disease (GERD).

But (and this is a big but) some heart patients may have chest pains that are very difficult to distinguish from reflux. Certainly, anytime you have chest pain, particularly if activity makes it worse, you should see your doctor. No waiting around.

Chapter 21

Ten Heartburn Web Sites

*T*he Internet is the world's biggest medical encyclopedia, covering everything from *alpha* (the first letter in the Greek alphabet and the first entry in my medical dictionary) to *ZZ* (the abbreviation for the genetic makeup of a person likely to develop chronic obstructive pulmonary disease or emphysema).

The trick, of course, is to be certain that the people who maintain the Web site you're clicking through have the Right Stuff. No fads, no fakes, just solid, reliable information.

As any reader of a *For Dummies* book knows, this chapter nominates ten of the best sites on the book's subject. Well, actually more than ten. Several top Web sites have their own favorite lists of links — some of which I simply couldn't resist. In the end, I ended up with 11. Or maybe 12.

Nonetheless, I am absolutely certain that I missed at least one somewhere in Cyberspace, so when you come across a site you find particularly useful, let me know. Perhaps we can add it to the next edition of this book. In the meantime, ladies and gentlemen: The envelopes, please!

The National Heartburn Alliance

www.heartburnalliance.org

The National Heartburn Alliance (NHBA) is a relatively new kid on the gastro-intestinal block. The Alliance created this site in 2000 to provide a support community for people with heartburn, educate ordinary folk about the causes and effects of this pain in the gut, offer solutions to relieve the ache, and generally improve the quality of life for people with reflux.

NHBA's user-friendly site serves this high-minded goal well, and it's reliable enough to have scored a featured link on the National Institute of Diabetes and Digestive and Kidney Diseases (NIDDK) site — which you can find later in this chapter.

NHBA offers online advice from the experts, self-care tips, food for thought (not to mention guidance on food for a healthy body), and statistics on heartburn so up-to-date that I use them throughout this book.

For technophobes who prefer a live voice at the end of a telephone, NHBA has a toll-free number: 877-471-2081.

International Foundation for Functional Gastrointestinal Disorders

www.iffgd.org

The International Foundation for Functional Gastrointestinal Disorders (IFFGD) specializes in clear information on how to recognize, diagnose, treat, and — not so incidentally — live with gastrointestinal disorders, including heartburn and GERD. Check out their treasure trove of heartburn facts and recommendations.

IFFGD is the lead organization in the Coalition Against Acid Reflux Disease (CAARD), an umbrella group of GERD-related professional and lay organizations with its very own toll-free number (888-964-2001). IFFGD is also the proud parent of GERD Awareness Week, created in November 1999 and celebrated (okay, marked) every year since.

HelpHeartburn.com

www.helpheartburn.com

GERD Information Center

www.gerd.com

Each of these two sites draws funding from a different pharmaceutical corporation. HelpHeartburn.com is the brainchild of Healthology, a company that puts together expert-based health sites with nonrestricted corporate grants. (**Translation:** The grant giver can't tell the grant getter what to do with the money). For example, Johnson & Johnson funds HelpHeartburn.com. There's no middleman at the GERD Information Center, a Web site created by Astra/Zeneca, an international drug company that makes two of the biggest-selling heartburn medications: Prilosec and Nexium.

Skeptics may find these situations disquieting, but the hard fact is that despite their corporate ties, both sites provide valuable links to online scientific libraries. Both sites provide access to tons of articles on the subject at hand, and unless you have a medical library in your living room, you'll have a hard time duplicating either of these lists of recent writing about heartburn and GERD.

In other words, don't let your potential bias get in the way of finding the news you need. If what you turn up on these sites helps you, use it. If the site sounds like a commercial, move on.

The American Gastroenterological Association

www.gastro.org

The 12,000-member American Gastroenterological Association (AGA), founded in 1897, is the oldest nonprofit specialty medical society in the United States.

So it's no surprise that the AGA Web site is chockablock with info about digestive disease symptoms, treatments, research initiatives, continuing medical education, practice management, medical position statements, and public policy information.

Unless you're planning to open your own medical practice, you can obviously pass by most of the links and head straight for the link regarding patients and the public. One click here brings up a wealth of goodies: a resource center, a magazine, a message board, a library, and a news bureau.

The American College of Gastroenterology

www.acg.gi.org

The American College of Gastroenterology (ACG), another group of folks who specialize in treating your digestive tract, has a different inducement. On the homepage, choose the Patient Information link. and then head to the section on GERD. There, in addition to some good information, you can find an offer for a totally free full-color video on acid reflux. Your only assignment, if you choose to accept it, is to fill out an address form and answer a few questions about your experience with GERD.

American Society for Gastrointestinal Endoscopy (ASGE)

www.asge.org

If your doctor suggests *endoscopy* (a diagnostic technique described in detail in Chapter 9), the American Society for Gastrointestinal Endoscopy (ASGE) Web site's specialized approach can help you wind your way through what may otherwise be an impermeable maze. After all, who else gives you the lowdown on a hot topic like how endoscopists reduce the risk of infection during an endoscopic procedure?

To unlock the site, go to the homepage and choose the link dedicated to patients and the public. When the screen changes, the patient information link provides numerous subcategories, including endoscopic procedures (a really clear chart with definitions) and one of those ever-popular doctor-shopping guides (by geographic area).

I hope you never need this site. But if you do, the trip is worth the clicks.

North American Society for Pediatric Gastroenterology, Hepatology and Nutrition

www.naspghan.org

True to its name, NASPGHAN — no, I can't pronounce it, and, no, I won't write out that whole title more than once, thank you! — has designed a Web site with both parents and kids in mind.

To enter, choose the link dedicated to the general public. Then choose the public information link, and scroll down to the GERD section. Your reward? Two age-related brochures — one for parents of infants and one for parents of teens.

Also check out a NASPGHAN offspring, the Children' Digestive Health and Nutrition Foundation. This organization has two Web sites designed for either very young kids (www.kidsacidreflux.org) or teenagers (www.teensacidreflux.org) to use. In each case, the site is age-appropriate. Any computer-literate kid can just click and go.

American Academy of Family Physicians

http://familydoctor.org

Aha! Did you notice something missing from that Web address? Right: No "www." But you do find plenty of the sort of down-home, friendly advice you'd expect from your family doctor. To reach the heartburn info, type "heartburn" into the search box on the homepage to get reassuring messages in English and Spanish. Some subjects look familiar, like *Hints on Dealing With the Discomfort,* for example. Some subjects are a tad more esoteric, like the description of a possible link between heartburn and asthma (the irritation of the first may trigger a flare-up of the second) or iron pills and heartburn (the pills upset your stomach and, bingo!)

With nobody pushing you to move along, the site makes you feel kind of like you have a doctor who makes house calls.

The American Dietetic Association

www.eatright.org

As you may expect, the American Dietetic Association (ADA) Web site is filled to bursting with food and diet tips, guidelines, research, policy, and stats. A search for "heartburn" turns up easy-to-read, practical, recent scientific reports. For example, on the day I tried it, I got 11 responses, including a guide to heartburn-free snacking.

Like the gastroenterologists and the endoscopists, the dietitians are eager and willing to help you find one of their own. On the homepage, enter your zip code in the box marked "Find a nutrition professional." Up comes the ADA disclaimer to which you must agree. Click "I agree" at the bottom of the page, and you get a list of registered dietitians right in your own neighborhood.

The Food and Drug Administration

www.fda.gov

The Food and Drug Administration (FDA) is America's first line of defense in protecting the safety of medical drugs and devices, and the agency shares with the United States Department of Agriculture (USDA) the task of protecting food.

To accomplish this humongous job, the FDA created an appropriately humongous Web site. For you health and nutrition junkies, when you enter the FDA's domain, you open the door to the world's biggest toy store. There's so much stuff on the (virtual) shelves that you hardly know which to grab first.

Luckily, in this store, all the toys are free. And what with cross-referencing and switching back and forth from one subject to another, you could linger here happily for days. Weeks. Years. Maybe forever. But time's a wastin'.

For people with heartburn, you can find the main event in the pages and pages and pages and . . . well, we'll settle for *many, many* pages of bulletins on drug approvals, drug problems, drug trials, drug development, reports, statistics, and opinions on heartburn/reflux/GERD.

Type any one of those words you know so well — *heartburn, GERD,* or *reflux* — into the search box on the homepage, and it's all yours. Best (worst?) of all, the FDA is continually updating its material, so when you come up for air, you can start all over again. Arrgh!

Chapter 22

Ten Sometimes Painful, Often Annoying, but Almost Never Fatal Digestive Disorders

- -

In This Chapter

▶ Figuring out when appendicitis is really a problem

▶ Understanding why your bowels treat you so badly

▶ Identifying an old (really old!) antidote that may actually work

▶ Naming the cause of a bad smell

▶ Getting all choked up

▶ Finding relief for hemorrhoids

▶ Placing inflammatory bowel diseases on the world map

- -

All kinds of troublemakers love to target the digestive tract.

This chapter title says *ten* disorders, but if you've read a *For Dummies* book before, you know how terrible these chapters are at sticking to that number. In this chapter, you see nine common pains in the gut, but you get ten because I combine "Constipation and Diarrhea" as one entry.

Luckily, although these conditions are all annoying, uncomfortable, or painful, modern medicine can cure or relieve them. And for more on the conditions that can rattle your innards, check out Chapter 1. Meanwhile, as my grandma Gloria-Don't-Call-Me-Gussie used to say, "Listen, it could always be worse."

Appendicitis

Appendicitis is a bacterial infection of the *appendix,* the sausage-shaped organ of no known value that hangs off your large intestine (or colon) in the lower-right corner of your abdomen.

The typical symptoms of an infected appendix are pain in the area your doctor calls the "lower right quadrant" (to the right and down from your belly button), plus a slight fever, an elevated white blood count (*white blood cells,* the body's shock troops, multiply to battle invading microorganisms), loss of appetite, nausea, vomiting, and constipation.

Appendicitis is more common among people living in the United States and Western Europe than in developing countries, suggesting a link to diet and/or activity levels (exercise to you). It's equally common among men and women except for a strange period between puberty and age 25 or 30 when the ratio of patients, at least in the United States, is three males for every two females.

Until late in the 19th century, when doctors discovered that they could cure appendicitis surgically, most people with appendicitis died of *peritonitis,* an infection of the lining of the body cavity caused by a burst appendix. Thanks to modern medicine, doctors diagnose appendicitis (by its primary symptoms or maybe a CT scan) and remove the appendix, and the patient returns to a healthy life.

Unfortunately, a surprising number of the appendixes that surgeons yank out are actually healthy organs. In 1997, the Nationwide Inpatient Sample of the Health Care Utilization Project reported this result for nearly 40,000 of the 261,134 appendectomies performed in the United States that year. The mistakes occurred more frequently in women, children younger than 5, and seniors older than 60, leading researchers to emphasize "the importance of developing more effective diagnostic strategies in the management of presumed appendicitis."

Bezoar

A *bezoar* (pronounced *bee*-zor) is a small chunk of hair or veggie gunk that has solidified in the digestive tract due to decreased motility of the gut (failure to move food along quickly), a situation that sometimes accompanies significant obesity, diabetes, or stomach surgery.

Doctors may mistake a bezoar that shows up on an MRI or CT scan for a tumor. As a rule, most bezoars don't cause any symptoms, but occasionally some may cause nausea, vomiting, pain, and bleeding. Bezoars of hair may require surgery; veggie bezoars rarely do.

Perhaps the most interesting thing about bezoars is their history as magical antidotes for certain poisons. For centuries, you'd dispatch your enemies by sprinkling something nasty, like arsenic, into their dinner wine. To protect yourself in potentially hostile company, you dropped a bezoar extracted from the stomach of a *ruminant* — an animal such as a goat or a cow that has more than one stomach — into your wineglass.

Believe it or not, recent studies at the century-old Scripps Institution of Oceanography in San Diego say that this maneuver may have worked — at least with arsenic, whose toxic constituents stick to sulfur compounds, like those in the hair proteins in a bezoar. Who knew?

Constipation and Diarrhea

The members of this dynamic/nondynamic duo are opposites in virtually every way. *Constipation* is almost always a mechanical problem, a failure of the intestinal tract to move food along efficiently. *Diarrhea* is often linked to an infection, a medicine, a food, or an emotional response that sends the intestines into overdrive.

Although constipation and diarrhea are uncomfortable and annoying, you can usually treat them with simple remedies, like more dietary fiber (constipation) or less of whatever irritates the gut (diarrhea).

Remember, though, both constipation and diarrhea are symptoms, not diseases. In worst-case scenarios, constipation may be a sign of an intestinal blockage, and diarrhea may be caused by potentially lethal food poisoning. If your discomfort persists or your symptoms are immediately severe, check with your doctor before self-medicating.

Gas (Flatulence)

Intestinal gas is the inevitable product of digestion's chemical reactions that release carbon dioxide, but the vast majority of gastrointestinal gas actually comes from air that you swallow. In fact, if you analyze intestinal gas (now, that's quite a job), its chemical composition is very close to that of the air you breathe.

Another source of gas is the resident population of intestinal bacteria that digest and ferment carbohydrates, like dietary fiber and the notorious beans immortalized in Mel Brooks's *Blazing Saddles.* After eating, these guys let loose hydrogen, carbon dioxide, and smelly methane gas.

You get rid of this gas by belching, breathing it out through your lungs, or expelling it from your intestinal tract. One study — imagine! a study on gas! — shows the average incidence of flatulence to be 13 to 21 times a day for a healthy adult male.

For most people, intestinal gas is no big deal, but *excess gas* troubles some. Defining how much is too much is pretty subjective, though. One man's excess gas may be another's fast belch.

If your gas comes with pain, weight loss, and other digestive symptoms, check it out with your doctor before self-medicating.

Defining a rude verb

How rude is the verb *to fart?* So rude, it seems, that the word is nowhere to be found in the classic 12-pound, 3,210-page *Webster's New American Dictionary of the English Language* (1941), or the semi-classic *Webster's New Collegiate Dictionary* (1957), or the contemporary pocket-size *Merriam-Webster Dictionary* (1997), or even the 26th edition of *Stedman's Medical Dictionary.* (But surprise! *Webster's New World College Dictionary,* 4th Edition, published in 1999, has the verb — huzzah.)

English authors have known and used the verb for at least the 600 years since Geoffrey Chaucer penned *The Canterbury Tales* in 1386. In fact, you may have come across some of the following examples listed. And for the truly curious, *The Random House Historical Dictionary of American Slang* (Volume 1, 1994) defines many fart-based nouns, adjectives, and verbs — a veritable cornucopia of really rude words, such as

- **To fart fire:** to show anger

- **To fart through silk:** describes the behavior of a person who lives in luxury

- **To fart around:** to waste time

- **To fart away:** to squander your resources

- **To fart off:** to ignore your responsibilities

Globus Sensation

Imagine these situations: You're about to stand up to give a report at the department meeting, the movie you're watching comes to a really scary part, or your best friend tells you how much you mean to him. And suddenly you're *all choked up*.

If you get choked up often enough, you may begin to wonder if something serious is going on. After your doctor excludes such unpleasant possibilities as esophageal spasms, reflux, *myasthenia gravis* (progressive loss of muscle power), or a tumor in your neck or throat, what's left is *globus*, a stress-related lump in the throat.

Doctors don't have a medical treatment for globus, but understanding the emotional link may help relieve the stress.

Hemorrhoids

Hemorrhoids may park at the end of the intestinal line, but doctors still classify them as a digestive problem.

External hemorrhoids are *varicosed* (or swollen) veins outside the ring of muscles around the anus; internal hemorrhoids are varicosed veins underneath the mucous membrane lining of the rectum.

Both external and internal hemorrhoids can be painful when moving your bowels. Warm baths may soothe the discomfort, and stool softeners may help make bowel movements feel a little less unpleasant.

Hemorrhoids sometimes bleed. If you have repeated bleeding, severe pain, or badly swollen hemorrhoids, check with your doctor to rule out any problems that may be more serious.

A gastrointestinal riddle

Hemorrhoids are sometimes called *piles*. So why is *pile* a synonym for *hemorrhoid*? Because the word *pile* comes from *pila*, Latin for *ball* (in this case the small ball-like swelling of a varicose vein at the rectum). One pile equals one hemorrhoid. Two piles equal two hemorrhoids. Lots of piles equal lots of hemorrhoids. Ouch.

Hiccups

What's a hiccup? Well, imagine an involuntary spasm happens in your *diaphragm* (the muscular band under your lungs) at the same time that your *glottis* (the opening from your mouth into your throat) closes involuntarily. When the glottis snaps shut, no air can flow down into your throat. Instead, it rushes out through your mouth — a hiccup.

Hiccups may simply be a reaction to swallowing unusually hot or spicy food, or they may be triggered by a medical condition. Abdominal surgery, a bladder infection, liver disease, and pancreatitis all irritate the vagus nerve that controls the diaphragm, thus causing hiccups.

Most of the time, the familiar home remedy of breathing into a paper bag can stop hiccups. Breathing into the paper bag increases the level of carbon dioxide in your blood, sending a signal to your brain to alert your lungs to take a deep breath, which stretches your diaphragm and ends the spasms. Drinking from the wrong side of a glass or getting someone to scare you can work because both force you to — gasp! — hold your breath for a second or two, an act that stops the motion of the diaphragm.

From time to time, however, hiccups go on and on and on and — well, you get the picture. The world's record remains with Iowan Charles Osborne, who started hiccupping in 1922 and kept it up for 69 years and five months. A hiccup every 1.5 seconds until 1990, when he suddenly stopped for no apparent reason.

Today, in such severe cases, doctors may recommend you have surgery to cut the vagus nerve, but Osborne died in 1991 with his vagus nerve intact and quiet as a lamb.

Irritable Bowel Syndrome (IBS)

IBS, commonly known as *nervous stomach,* is a motor disorder of the entire gastrointestinal tract. Translation: Your gut, from stomach to colon, goes into hyperdrive, triggering abdominal pain and bloating, plus diarrhea and/or constipation.

No one knows the causes of IBS. Some people blame their IBS on stress. Others point to their sensitivity to certain foods. But people with IBS — who are generally healthy, otherwise — may experience symptoms with or without emotional turmoil and regardless of what they eat.

Nonetheless, just as the eyes are the window to the soul, the intestines are the mirror of the mind. Relieving stress — including the stress of assuming you have some other digestive disease or condition — may help alleviate IBS.

If IBS comes with constipation, adding dietary fiber may be useful; vice versa for people whose IBS appears as diarrhea. In severe cases of IBS, doctors may prescribe antispasmodic drugs to calm jumpy gastro muscles or antidepressants, which not only soothe the mind but also ease intestinal pain.

Inflammatory Bowel Disease (IBD)

Inflammatory bowel disease is an umbrella term for several chronic inflammations of the gastrointestinal tract, most often Crohn's disease (CD) and ulcerative colitis (UC).

Although both are inflammatory conditions, CD and UC are different in many respects. For example:

- Ulcerative colitis only occasionally causes pain, doesn't respond to antibiotics, and occurs more commonly in nonsmokers than in smokers.

- Crohn's disease frequently causes pain, responds to antibiotics but may recur after surgery, and occurs more commonly in smokers than in nonsmokers.

Nobody knows exactly what causes either CD or UC, but genetics seems to play a role. So both conditions may run in families. One in six patients with IBD has a close relative with the same problem, and a child with two IBD parents has about a one-in-three chance of developing CD or UC. Ethnicity may also be a factor in the occurrence of IBD. It's most common in the United States, Great Britain, Norway, and Sweden, and it's least common in southern Europe, Asia, Africa, and South America. Table 22-1 shows the geographical distribution of IBD.

Table 22-1	Finding IBD Patients	
Geographic Areas	*Number of Cases per 100,000 People*	
	Ulcerative Colitis	*Crohn's Disease*
United States/United Kingdom	11	7
Southern Europe/Southern Africa/Australia	2	6.3
Asia/South America	0.5	0.1

Source: Eugene Braunwald, et al., Harrison's Principles of Internal Medicine, 15th ed. (New York: McGraw Hill, 2001)

Table 22-2 lists self-help groups — a good resource for those of you who have, or know someone who has, IBD.

Table 22-2	Finding Help for IBD
Group	*Toll-Free Number*
Crohn's and Colitis Foundation of America	800-387-1479
Crohn's and Colitis Foundation of Canada	800-932-2423
National Association for Colitis and Crohn's Disease (U.K.)	0845-130-2233

Glossary

. . . .

Making your way through most books about a medical condition can be challenging. All the terms can become confusing. With this title, in true *For Dummies* fashion, I've tried to make things as simple as possible for you by providing explanations that don't leave you scratching your head. But should you need a quick refresher on heartburn-related terms, whether you're reading this book or other information about heartburn and reflux, this section is a short but useful dictionary that pulls most of the medical words in *Heartburn & Reflux For Dummies* into one neat glossary.

Note: Any word printed in **italic and bold type** has its own definition in its own rightful alphabetical place in this glossary.

Abdomen: The area between the chest and pelvis, roughly from waist to about two inches below the navel.

Achalasia: Weakness of the esophageal muscles. People with achalasia are unable to push food along efficiently from mouth to stomach.

Acid: The opposite of *base* (noun) or ***basic*** (adjective). The terms acid and base are used to describe ***pH,*** a scale used to measure the acidity of a water-based solution.

Acid perfusion test: A diagnostic test for reflux that assesses the sensitivity of the esophageal lining to an acid solution.

Acid reflux: Another term for ***reflux.***

Acid suppressor: Medicine that reduces the normal secretion of acidic stomach juices. See ***histamine (H2) blockers, proton pump inhibitors.***

Adverse effects: Unexpected, unusual, infrequent, and possibly serious reactions to medicines.

Ambulatory 24-hour pH monitoring: A procedure that measures the acidity of the liquids in the esophagus over a full day.

Antacids: Compounds that neutralize acid solutions. Saliva is a natural antacid; baking soda (sodium bicarbonate) is a chemical antacid.

Antireflux surgery: See ***fundoplication.***

Bariatrician: A physician specializing in health issues related to weight.

Barium swallow: A test during which the patient swallows a thick solution containing the element barium. The solution coats the esophageal lining, making abnormalities such as an *esophageal stricture* visible on X-ray.

Barrett's esophagus: A precancerous change in cells lining the esophagus.

Basic: The modern term for the opposite of acid. Base and basic replace the outmoded terms alkali and alkaline.

Bernstein test: See *acid perfusion test.*

Bloat: A feeling of fullness due to the presence of air in the digestive system.

Body mass index (BMI): A description of weight relative to height. The ratio is expressed in a number, such as 24, that serves as a predictor of your risk for weight-related illnesses including reflux.

Bolus: The easy-to-swallow mass created when saliva-moistened food is mashed and compacted in the mouth.

Bougie: An instrument used to dilate a constricted esophagus.

Chyme: The thick mass produced when your stomach begins to digest food.

Colic: An outmoded term for *reflux* symptoms in infants.

Diaphragm: The large muscle that divides the chest from the abdomen.

Diaphragmatic hiatus: The opening in the diaphragm through which the esophagus passes to enter the stomach.

Digestion: The process by which the body breaks food down into its component parts (for example protein, fat, carbohydrates, vitamins, minerals, and other nutrients).

Digestive system: The organs and glands used to digest food: Mouth, esophagus, stomach, small intestine, large intestine, liver, pancreas, gallbladder.

Digestive tract: The tubelike structure that begins at the mouth and ends at the anus.

Duodenum: The top of the *small intestine,* where food enters from the stomach.

Dysphasia: Difficulty in swallowing.

Endoscope: A flexible instrument that enables a doctor to look inside the body or into a tube such as the *esophagus.*

Esophageal dilation: A procedure that stretches an esophagus narrowed by repeated exposure to *reflux.*

Esophageal erosion: An injury to the esophageal lining caused by long-term exposure to acid *reflux* that may lead to an *ulcer* (an open sore).

Esophageal manometry: A test that measures the strength of the esophageal muscles.

Esophageal spasms: Muscle contractions that temporarily narrow the esophagus and prevent swallowing.

Esophageal stricture: Narrowing of the esophagus due to damaged tissues.

Esophagitis: Irritation of the esophagus.

Esophagus: The approximately 8-inch tube that carries food from the *pharynx* to the stomach. Also known as the throat.

Fundoplication: A surgical procedure during which the top of the stomach is folded around the bottom of the esophagus, tightening the *lower esophageal sphincter* and reducing the risk of *reflux.*

Gastric juices: The acid secretions released by the stomach and other organs such as the pancreas. Gastric juices are required for digesting food.

Gastroenterologist: A physician specializing in disorders of the *digestive tract.*

Gastroesophageal flap valve: Folds of tissue at the entrance from the *esophagus* to the *stomach.*

Gastroesophageal junction: The place in the *digestive tract* where the esophagus meets the stomach.

Gastroesophageal reflux disease (GERD): A medical condition characterized by chronic and frequent *reflux. Note:* In Britain, esophagus is spelled oesophagus, so GERD becomes GORD.

Gastrointestinal tract: The *digestive tract.*

GERD: See *gastroesophageal reflux disease.*

GI series: X-ray examination of the *gastrointestinal tract.*

GI tract: Abbreviation for *gastrointestinal tract.*

Gullet: Synonym for *esophagus.*

Heartburn: The pain associated with *reflux.* Although the pain is felt in the center of the chest, where the heart is normally located, heartburn has no relation to the heart.

Hiatal hernia: A small bulge of the stomach through a gap in the *diaphragm* at the place where the *esophagus* passes through.

Histamine (H2) blockers: Compounds whose molecules attach to specific sites (receptors) on the cells in the walls of the intestinal tract, thereby preventing a substance called histamine from stimulating the secretion of stomach acids.

Interaction: The reaction that may occur between two or more chemical compounds, such as two medicines.

Laparoscope: A rigid tube containing a miniature television camera. Laparoscopes are used for viewing internal parts of the body such as the *esophagus.*

Laparoscopic surgery: An operation in which the surgical field is viewed through a laparoscope inserted into a narrow tube called a *trocar,* and the procedure is performed with specialized small instruments inserted through additional trocars, each of which requires only a ½ to 1-inch incision.

Large intestine: The lower part of the *digestive tract,* an area known as the colon where waste is squeezed dry and compacted into feces, which is then pushed down into the *rectum* and out through the anus.

Larynx: The "voice box," or the organ that enables you to talk.

Lower esophageal sphincter (LES): The muscle that controls the opening between the *esophagus* and the *stomach.* When the lower esophageal sphincter doesn't stay closed after food has passed through, acid and stomach contents may reflux back into the esophagus.

Lower GI series: A radiological examination of the lower part of the *gastrointestinal tract,* including the colon and the rectum. Also know as a *barium enema.*

Manometry: See *esophageal manometry.*

Metabolism: The process by which your body extracts nutrients from food and uses the nutrients as energy or building materials for tissues and chemicals such as enzymes is metabolism.

Nissen fundoplication: See *fundoplication.*

Nonsteroidal anti-inflammatory drugs (NSAIDs, pronounced en-seds): Medicines which relief pain and reduce inflammation. Examples include aspirin, ibuprofen, and naproxen.

OTC: The abbreviation for over the counter, a term applied to medicines available without a prescription.

Otolaryngologist: A physician who specializes in disorders of the ear, nose, and throat (sometimes abbreviated as ENT).

Peristalsis: The muscular contractions of the walls of the digestive tract that propel food down the esophagus, into and out of the stomach, on through the intestines, and eventually out of the body.

pH: A number on a scale used to measure the acidity of a water-based solution such as household ammonia, black coffee, and the gastric juices. The higher the number, the more *basic* the solution. The lower the number, the more acid the solution.

Pharynx: The opening at the back of the mouth that opens into the *esophagus.*

Proton pump inhibitors (PPIs): Medicines that block the ability of special cells in your stomach wall to release stomach acids. PPIs also appear to help heal reflux-related esophageal injuries.

Pulmonologist: A physician specializing in disorders of the respiratory system.

Pyrosis: The medical term for *heartburn,* from *pyro,* the Latin word for *fire.*

Radiologist: A physician specializing in the use of radiology (x-rays) to diagnose and treat disease.

Rectum: The last section of the *large intestine,* the area from which waste is expelled through the anus.

Reflux: The flow of acid stomach liquids back through the *lower esophageal sphincter* into the *esophagus.* Used as both a noun and a verb, as in "Acid reflux from the stomach may reflux back into the esophagus."

Regurgitation: The flow of actual food backwards from the stomach into the *esophagus.*

Saliva: A watery, naturally *basic* liquid secreted by the salivary glands.

Scintigraphy: A computerized radiological scan sometimes used to track the passage of food through the stomach of a child too young for other *reflux* diagnostic exams.

Side effects: Normal, totally expected consequences of taking a medicine.

Small intestine: A 20-foot–long, coiled tube in your abdomen that extracts proteins, fats, carbohydrates, vitamins, minerals, and other nutrients from food and then sends them off to be used for energy or as building blocks for new tissue.

Sphincter: A ring of muscle, such as the *lower esophageal sphincter*.

Stomach: The pouchy part of the digestive tube located on the left side of the body above the waist and behind the ribs. The muscles circling the stomach break food into ever smaller pieces as glands in the stomach walls release "stomach juices" — a rich, highly acidic blend of enzymes, hydrochloric acid (HCl), and mucus, which begin the digestion of proteins and fats into their constituent building blocks, amino acids, and fatty acids.

Stricture: A narrowing of a tube such as the *esophagus.*

Trachea: The "wind pipe," a tube that carries air into the lungs when you breathe.

Transient LES relaxations: Accidental openings of the lower esophageal sphincter that make belching/burping possible, thus expelling excess air from the stomach.

Trochar: A tube through which a medical instrument such as a *laparoscope* is inserted into the body.

Ulcer: An injury on the surface of skin or mucous membranes. A peptic ulcer is an injury on the surface of the lining of the *stomach* or the *duodenum.*

Upper esophageal sphincter: A muscular ring at the back of the mouth at the entrance to the esophagus.

Upper GI series: A series of X-ray pictures of the upper part of the gastrointestinal tract, including the *esophagus* and *stomach.*

Water brash: A rush of saliva that fills the mouth and flows down the *esophagus* as a natural reaction to the presence of acidic stomach liquids during *reflux.*

Index

●●

• B •

• *M* •

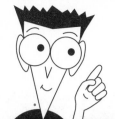

FOR DUMMIES®

The easy way to get more done and have more fun

PERSONAL FINANCE & BUSINESS

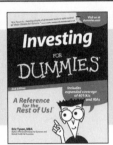

Investing FOR DUMMIES
2nd Edition
A Reference for the Rest of Us!
0-7645-2431-3

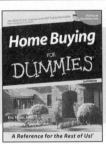

Home Buying FOR DUMMIES
2nd Edition
A Reference for the Rest of Us!
0-7645-5331-3

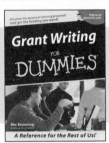

Grant Writing FOR DUMMIES
A Reference for the Rest of Us!
0-7645-5307-0

Also available:

Accounting For Dummies
(0-7645-5314-3)

Business Plans Kit For
Dummies
(0-7645-5365-8)

Managing For Dummies
(1-5688-4858-7)

Mutual Funds For Dummies
(0-7645-5329-1)

QuickBooks All-in-One Desk
Reference For Dummies
(0-7645-1963-8)

Resumes For Dummies
(0-7645-5471-9)

Small Business Kit For
Dummies
(0-7645-5093-4)

Starting an eBay Business
For Dummies
(0-7645-1547-0)

Taxes For Dummies 2003
(0-7645-5475-1)

HOME, GARDEN, FOOD & WINE

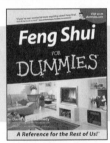

Feng Shui FOR DUMMIES
A Reference for the Rest of Us!
0-7645-5295-3

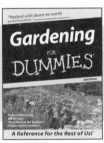

Gardening FOR DUMMIES
2nd Edition
A Reference for the Rest of Us!
0-7645-5130-2

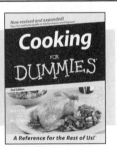

Cooking FOR DUMMIES
2nd Edition
A Reference for the Rest of Us!
0-7645-5250-3

Also available:

Bartending For Dummies
(0-7645-5051-9)

Christmas Cooking For
Dummies
(0-7645-5407-7)

Cookies For Dummies
(0-7645-5390-9)

Diabetes Cookbook For
Dummies
(0-7645-5230-9)

Grilling For Dummies
(0-7645-5076-4)

Home Maintenance For
Dummies
(0-7645-5215-5)

Slow Cookers For Dummies
(0-7645-5240-6)

Wine For Dummies
(0-7645-5114-0)

FITNESS, SPORTS, HOBBIES & PETS

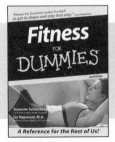

Fitness FOR DUMMIES
2nd Edition
Suzanne Schlosberg
Liz Neporent, M.A.
A Reference for the Rest of Us!
0-7645-5167-1

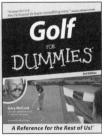

Golf FOR DUMMIES
2nd Edition
Gary McCord
A Reference for the Rest of Us!
0-7645-5146-9

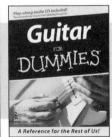

Guitar FOR DUMMIES
Play-along audio CD included!
A Reference for the Rest of Us!
0-7645-5106-X

Also available:

Cats For Dummies
(0-7645-5275-9)

Chess For Dummies
(0-7645-5003-9)

Dog Training For Dummies
(0-7645-5286-4)

Labrador Retrievers For
Dummies
(0-7645-5281-3)

Martial Arts For Dummies
(0-7645-5358-5)

Piano For Dummies
(0-7645-5105-1)

Pilates For Dummies
(0-7645-5397-6)

Power Yoga For Dummies
(0-7645-5342-9)

Puppies For Dummies
(0-7645-5255-4)

Quilting For Dummies
(0-7645-5118-3)

Rock Guitar For Dummies
(0-7645-5356-9)

Weight Training For Dummies
(0-7645-5168-X)

Available wherever books are sold.
Go to www.dummies.com or call 1-877-762-2974 to order direct

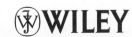

WILEY

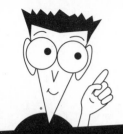
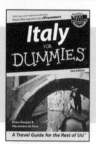
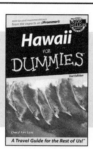
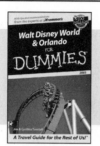
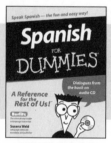
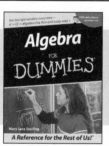
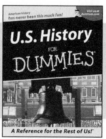
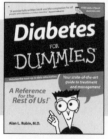
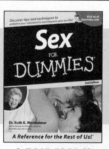
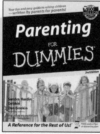

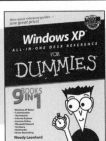
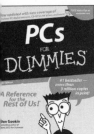
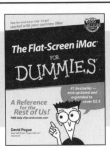
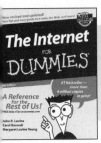
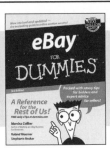
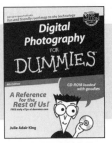
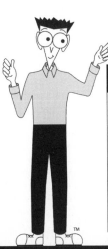
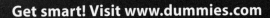

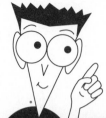

FOR DUMMIES®

Helping you expand your horizons and realize your potential

GRAPHICS & WEB SITE DEVELOPMENT

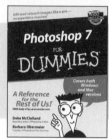 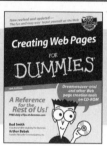 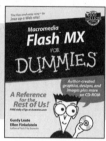

Photoshop 7 For Dummies
0-7645-1651-5

Creating Web Pages For Dummies
0-7645-1643-4

Macromedia Flash MX For Dummies
0-7645-0895-4

Also available:

Adobe Acrobat 5 PDF For Dummies (0-7645-1652-3)

ASP.NET For Dummies (0-7645-0866-0)

ColdFusion MX For Dummies (0-7645-1672-8)

Dreamweaver MX For Dummies (0-7645-1630-2)

FrontPage 2002 For Dummies (0-7645-0821-0)

HTML 4 For Dummies (0-7645-0723-0)

Illustrator 10 For Dummies (0-7645-3636-2)

PowerPoint 2002 For Dummies (0-7645-0817-2)

Web Design For Dummies (0-7645-0823-7)

PROGRAMMING & DATABASES

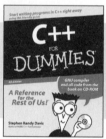 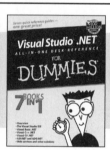 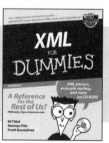

C++ For Dummies
0-7645-0746-X

Visual Studio .NET All-in-One Desk Reference For Dummies
0-7645-1626-4

XML For Dummies
0-7645-1657-4

Also available:

Access 2002 For Dummies (0-7645-0818-0)

Beginning Programming For Dummies (0-7645-0835-0)

Crystal Reports 9 For Dummies (0-7645-1641-8)

Java & XML For Dummies (0-7645-1658-2)

Java 2 For Dummies (0-7645-0765-6)

JavaScript For Dummies (0-7645-0633-1)

Oracle9i For Dummies (0-7645-0880-6)

Perl For Dummies (0-7645-0776-1)

PHP and MySQL For Dummies (0-7645-1650-7)

SQL For Dummies (0-7645-0737-0)

Visual Basic .NET For Dummies (0-7645-0867-9)

LINUX, NETWORKING & CERTIFICATION

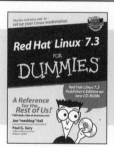 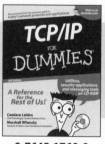 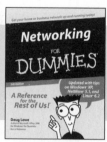

Red Hat Linux 7.3 For Dummies
0-7645-1545-4

TCP/IP For Dummies
0-7645-1760-0

Networking For Dummies
0-7645-0772-9

Also available:

A+ Certification For Dummies (0-7645-0812-1)

CCNP All-in-One Certification For Dummies (0-7645-1648-5)

Cisco Networking For Dummies (0-7645-1668-X)

CISSP For Dummies (0-7645-1670-1)

CIW Foundations For Dummies (0-7645-1635-3)

Firewalls For Dummies (0-7645-0884-9)

Home Networking For Dummies (0-7645-0857-1)

Red Hat Linux All-in-One Desk Reference For Dummies (0-7645-2442-9)

UNIX For Dummies (0-7645-0419-3)

Available wherever books are sold.
Go to www.dummies.com or call 1-877-762-2974 to order direct

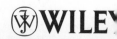

WILEY